Pocket Reference for

# ECGs
# MADE
# EASY

Barbara Aehlert, RN, BSPA
Southwest EMS Education, Inc.
Phoenix, AZ/Pursley, TX

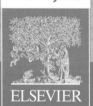

MOSBY JEMS

ELSEVIER

Fourth Edition

# MOSBY JEMS
## ELSEVIER

3251 Riverport Lane
Maryland Heights, Missouri 63043

POCKET REFERENCE FOR ECGs MADE EASY,     ISBN: 978-0-323-06928-1
FOURTH EDITION
**Copyright © 2011, 2006, 2002, 1995 by Mosby, Inc., an affiliate of Elsevier Inc.**

---

### Notice

---

ISBN: 978-0-323-06928-1

*Executive Editor:* Linda Honeycutt Dickison
*Associate Developmental Editor:*  Mary Jo Adams
*Publishing Services Manager:* Julie Eddy
*Senior Project Manager:* Andrea Campbell
*Design Direction:* Maggie Reid

Printed in China

Last digit is the print number:
9  8  7  6  5  4  3  2

Working together to grow
libraries in developing countries
www.elsevier.com | www.bookaid.org | www.sabre.org

ELSEVIER    BOOK AID International    Sabre Foundation

# Preface

The purpose of this pocket reference is to provide you with a handy, easy-to-use manual that is needed to interpret basic dysrhythmias. This reference is intended to accompany the *ECGs Made Easy* textbook. A brief description of each rhythm discussed in the textbook appears in this reference. Each description is accompanied by a summary of the characteristics of the rhythm and a sample rhythm strip. All rhythm strips were recorded in lead II unless otherwise noted. Possible patient signs and symptoms related to the rhythm and treatment options are included in the *ECGs Made Easy* textbook.

I hope you find this pocket reference of assistance, and I welcome your comments and suggestions.

Best regards,
Barbara Aehlert

# Acknowledgments

I would like to thank Andrew Baird, CEP; James Bratcher; Holly Button, CEP; Gretchen Chalmers, CEP; Thomas Cole, CEP; Brent Haines, CEP; Paul Honeywell, CEP; Timothy Klatt, RN; Bill Loughran, RN; Andrea Lowrey, RN; Joe Martinez, CEP; Stephanos Orphanidis, CEP; Jason Payne, CEP; Steve Ruehs, CEP; Patty Seneski, RN; David Stockton, CEP; Jason Stodghill, CEP; Dionne Socie, CEP; Kristina Tellez, CEP; and Fran Wojculewicz, RN, for providing many of the rhythm strips used in this text.

I would also like to thank the text reviewers for their comments and suggestions, which helped to improve the clarity of the information presented in this text.

# About the Author

Barbara Aehlert is the President of Southwest EMS Education, Inc., in Phoenix, Arizona, and Pursley, Texas. She has been a registered nurse for more than 30 years, with clinical experience in medical/surgical and critical care nursing, and she has more than 20 years experience in prehospital education. Barbara is an active CPR, First Aid, ACLS, and PALS instructor.

# Contents

# Anatomy and Physiology

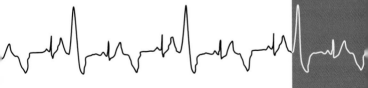

## LOCATION OF THE HEART

The heart is a hollow muscular organ that lies in the space between the lungs (mediastinum) in the middle of the chest. It sits behind the sternum and just above the diaphragm (Figure 1-1). Approximately two thirds of the heart lies to the left of the midline of the sternum. The remaining third lies to the right of the sternum.

The base of the heart is its upper portion and is formed mainly by the left atrium, with a small amount of right atrium. It lies at approximately the level of the second rib, immediately in front of the esophagus and descending aorta. The heart's apex, or lower portion, is formed by the tip of the left ventricle. The apex lies just above the diaphragm, between the fifth and sixth ribs, in the midclavicular line.

## HEART CHAMBERS

### Atria

The heart has four chambers (Figure 1-2). The two upper chambers are the right and left **atria**. The atria have thin walls. Their purpose is to *receive* blood. The right atrium receives blood low in oxygen from:

- The superior vena cava, which carries blood from the head and upper extremities

- The inferior vena cava, which carries blood from the lower body
- The coronary sinus, which is the largest vein that drains the heart

The left atrium receives freshly oxygenated blood from the lungs via the right and left pulmonary veins. The wall of the right atrium is about 2 mm thick and the wall of the left atrium is about 3 mm thick. Blood is pumped from the atria through an atrioventricular valve and into the ventricles.

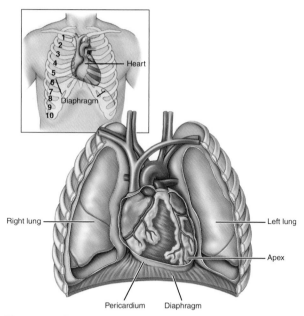

**Figure 1-1**    The heart lies in the space between the lungs (mediastinum) in the middle of the chest. It sits behind the sternum and just above the diaphragm.

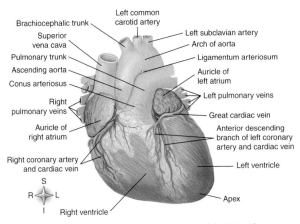

Brachiocephalic trunk
Superior vena cava
Pulmonary trunk
Ascending aorta
Conus arteriosus
Right pulmonary veins
Auricle of right atrium
Right coronary artery and cardiac vein

Left common carotid artery
Left subclavian artery
Arch of aorta
Ligamentum arteriosum
Auricle of left atrium
Left pulmonary veins
Great cardiac vein
Anterior descending branch of left coronary artery and cardiac vein
Left ventricle
Apex
Right ventricle

**Figure 1-2**   Anterior view of the heart and great vessels.

## Ventricles

The heart's two lower chambers are the right and left ventricles. The walls of the ventricles are much thicker than those of the atria. Their purpose is to pump blood. The right ventricle pumps blood to the lungs. The left ventricle pumps blood out to the body.

The right and left sides of the heart are separated by an internal wall of connective tissue called a septum. The interatrial septum separates the right and left atria. The interventricular septum separates the right and left ventricles (Figure 1-3, *A*). The septa separate the heart into two functional pumps. The right atrium and right ventricle make up one pump. The left atrium and left ventricle make up the other (Figure 1-3, *B*).

The job of the right side of the heart is to pump unoxygenated blood to and through the lungs to the left side of the heart. This is called the *pulmonary circulation*. The right side of the heart is a low-pressure system. The left side of the heart is a high-pressure pump. The job of the left heart is to receive oxygenated blood and pump it out to the rest of the body. This is called the *systemic circulation*.

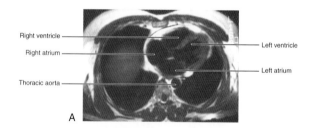

A

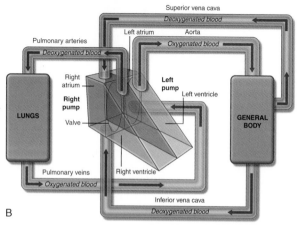

B

**Figure 1-3** **A,** Magnetic resonance image of the midthorax, showing the heart's chambers and septa. **B,** The heart has two functional pumps.

## SURFACES OF THE HEART

The front (anterior) surface of the heart lies behind the sternum and costal cartilages. It is formed by portions of the right atrium and the left and right ventricles. However, because the heart is tilted slightly toward the left in the chest, the right ventricle is the area of the heart that lies most directly behind the sternum. The heart's left side (left lateral surface) is made up mostly of the left ventricle. The heart's bottom (inferior) surface is formed by both the right and left ventricles. The inferior surface of the heart is also called the diaphragmatic surface. Figure 1-4 shows

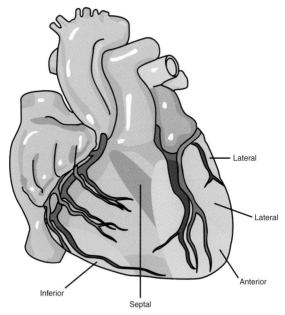

**Figure 1-4**    Surfaces of the heart. Posterior surface not shown.

the surfaces of the heart. Note that the posterior surface of the heart is not shown.

## LAYERS OF THE HEART

The walls of the heart are made up of three tissue layers: the endocardium, myocardium, and epicardium (Table 1-1). The heart's innermost layer is the endocardium. The endocardium is a thin, smooth layer of epithelium and connective tissue that lines the heart's inner chambers, valves, chordae tendineae, and papillary muscles. It is continuous with the innermost layer (tunica intima) of the arteries, veins, and capillaries of the body. This creates a continuous, closed circulatory system.

The myocardium (middle layer) is a thick, muscular layer that consists of cardiac muscle fibers (cells) responsible for the pumping action of the heart. The myocardium is subdivided

| Table **1-1** | Layers of the Heart Wall |
| --- | --- |
| **EPICARDIUM** | • External layer of the heart<br>• Coronary arteries, blood capillaries, lymph capillaries, nerve fibers, nerves, and fat are found in this layer |
| **MYOCARDIUM** | • Middle and thickest layer of the heart<br>• Responsible for heart's pumping action |
| **ENDOCARDIUM** | • Innermost layer of the heart<br>• Lines heart's inner chambers, valves, chordae tendineae, and papillary muscles<br>• Continuous with innermost layer of arteries, veins, and capillaries of body |

into two areas. The innermost half of the myocardium is called the subendocardial area because it lies below and the outermost half is called the subepicardial area. The muscle fibers of the myocardium are separated by connective tissues that have a rich supply of capillaries and nerve fibers.

The heart's outermost layer is called the epicardium. The epicardium is continuous with the inner lining of the pericardium at the heart's apex. The epicardium contains blood capillaries, lymph capillaries, nerve fibers, and fat. The main coronary arteries lie on the epicardial surface of the heart. They feed this area first before entering the myocardium and supplying the heart's inner layers with oxygenated blood.

The pericardium is a double-walled sac that encloses the heart and helps protect it from trauma and infection. The rough outer layer of the pericardial sac is called the *fibrous parietal pericardium*. It anchors the heart to some of the structures around it, such as the sternum and diaphragm. This helps prevent excessive movement of the heart in the chest with changes in body position. The inner layer, the *serous pericardium*, consists of two layers: parietal and visceral. The parietal layer lines the inside of the fibrous pericardium. The visceral layer (also called the epicardium) adheres to the outside of the heart and forms the outer layer of the heart muscle. Between the visceral and parietal layers is a space (the pericardial space) that normally contains about 20 mL of serous fluid. This fluid acts as a lubricant, preventing friction as the heart beats.

# CARDIAC MUSCLE

Cardiac muscle is found only in the heart. Cardiac muscle fibers make up the walls of the heart. These fibers have striations, or stripes, similar to that of skeletal muscle. Each muscle fiber is made up of many muscle cells. Each muscle cell is enclosed in a membrane called a sarcolemma. Within each cell are mitochondria, the energy-producing parts of a cell, and hundreds of long, tubelike structures called myofibrils. Myofibrils are made up of many sarcomeres, the basic protein units responsible for contraction. The process of contraction requires adenosine triphosphate (ATP) for energy. The mitochondria that are interspersed between the myofibrils are important sites of ATP production.

The sarcolemma has holes in it that lead into tubes called T (transverse) tubules. T-tubules are extensions of the cell membrane. Another system of tubules, the sarcoplasmic reticulum (SR), stores calcium. Muscle cells need calcium in order to contract. Calcium is moved from the sarcoplasm of the muscle cell into the sarcoplasmic reticulum by means of "pumps" in the sarcoplasmic reticulum.

There are certain places in the cell membrane where sodium (Na+), potassium (K+), and calcium (Ca++) can pass. These openings are called pores or channels. There are specific channels for sodium (sodium channels), potassium (potassium channels), and calcium (calcium channels). When the muscle is relaxed, the calcium channels are closed. As a result, calcium cannot pass through the membrane of the sarcoplasmic reticulum. This results in a high concentration of calcium in the sarcoplasmic reticulum and a low concentration in the sarcoplasm, where the muscle cells (sarcomeres) are found. If the muscle cells do not have calcium available to them, contraction is inhibited (the muscle is relaxed).

T-tubules pass completely through the sarcolemma and go around the muscle cells. The job of the T-tubules is to conduct impulses from the cell's surface (sarcolemma) down into the cell to the sarcoplasmic reticulum. When an impulse travels along the membrane of the sarcoplasmic reticulum, the calcium channels open. Calcium rapidly leaves the sarcoplasmic reticulum and enters the sarcoplasm. The muscle cells are then stimulated to contract.

Much of the calcium that enters the cell's sarcoplasm comes from the interstitial fluid surrounding the cardiac muscle cells through the T-tubules. This is important because without the extra calcium from the T-tubules, the strength of a cardiac muscle contraction would be considerably reduced. Thus, the force of cardiac muscle contraction depends largely on the concentration of calcium ions in the extracellular fluid.

Each sarcomere is composed of thin filaments and thick filaments. The thin filaments are made up of actin and actin-binding proteins. Actin-binding proteins include tropomyosin and troponin-T, troponin-C, and troponin-I, among others. The thick filaments are made up of hundreds of myosin molecules. Contraction occurs when the muscle is stimulated. Projections on the thin actin filaments interact with the thick myosin filaments and form crossbridges. The crossbridges use energy (ATP) to bend. This allows the actin filaments to slide over the myosin filaments toward the center of the sarcomere and overlap. This overlap causes shortening of the muscles cells, resulting in contraction. Actin-binding proteins hinder the formation of crossbridges with myosin. When crossbridge formation is hindered, the muscle is relaxed.

Cardiac muscle fibers are long branching cells that fit together tightly at junctions called *intercalated disks*. The arrangement of these tight-fitting junctions gives an appearance of a syncytium, that is, resembling a network of cells with no separation between the individual cells. The intercalated disks fit together in such a way that they form gap junctions. Gap junctions allow cells to communicate with each other. They function as electrical connections and permit the exchange of nutrients, metabolites, ions, and small molecules. As a result, an electrical impulse can be quickly conducted throughout the wall of a heart chamber. This characteristic allows the walls of both atria (likewise, the walls of both ventricles) to contract almost at the same time.

## HEART VALVES

The heart has a skeleton. The skeleton is made up of four rings of thick connective tissue. This tissue surrounds the bases of the pulmonary trunk, aorta, and the heart valves. The heart's skeleton helps form the partitions (septa) that separate the atria from the ventricles. It also provides secure attachments for the valves and chambers of the heart.

There are four valves in the heart: two sets of atrioventricular (AV) valves and two sets of semilunar (SL) valves (Table 1-2). Their purpose is to make sure blood flows in one direction through the heart's chambers and prevent the backflow of blood.

## Atrioventricular Valves

Atrioventricular (AV) valves separate the atria from the ventricles. The two AV valves consist of the following:

- Tough, fibrous rings (annuli fibrosi)
- Flaps (leaflets or cusps) of endocardium
- Chordae tendineae
- Papillary muscles

The tricuspid valve is the AV valve that lies between the right atrium and right ventricle. It consists of three separate cusps or flaps. It is larger in diameter and thinner than the mitral valve. The mitral (or bicuspid) valve has only two cusps. It lies between the left atrium and left ventricle.

As the atria fill with blood, the pressure within the atrial chamber rises. This pressure forces the tricuspid and mitral valves

| Table 1-2 | Heart Valves | | |
|---|---|---|---|
| Valve Type | Name | Right Heart vs. Left Heart | Location |
| Atrioventricular (AV) | Tricuspid | Right | Separates right atrium and right ventricle |
| | Mitral (Bicuspid) | Left | Separates left atrium and left ventricle |
| Semilunar | Pulmonic | Right | Between right ventricle and pulmonary artery |
| | Aortic | Left | Between left ventricle and aorta |

open. On the right side of the heart, blood low in oxygen empties into the right ventricle. On the left side of the heart, freshly oxygenated blood empties into the left ventricle. After the atria contract, the pressures in the atria and ventricles equalize, and the tricuspid and mitral valves partially close. The ventricles then contract (systole). This causes the pressure within the ventricles to rise sharply. The tricuspid and mitral valves close completely when the pressure within the ventricles exceeds that of the atria.

### Semilunar Valves

The pulmonic and aortic valves are semilunar (SL) valves. The semilunar valves prevent backflow of blood from the aorta and pulmonary arteries into the ventricles. The SL valves have three cusps shaped like half-moons. The openings of the SL valves are smaller than the openings of the AV valves. The flaps of the SL valves are smaller and thicker than the AV valves. Unlike the AV valves, the semilunar valves are not attached to chordae tendineae.

When the ventricles contract, the SL valves open, allowing blood to flow out of the ventricles. When the right ventricle contracts, blood low in oxygen flows through the pulmonic valve into the right and left pulmonary arteries. When the left ventricle contracts, freshly oxygenated blood flows through the aortic valve into the aorta and out to the body. The SL valves close as ventricular contraction ends and the pressure in the pulmonary artery and aorta exceeds that of the ventricles.

## HEART SOUNDS

Heart sounds occur because of vibrations in the tissues of the heart caused by the closing of the heart's valves. Vibrations are created as blood flow is suddenly increased or slowed with the contraction and relaxation of the heart chambers and with the opening and closing of the valves.

Normal heart sounds are called S1 and S2. The first heart sound ("lubb") occurs during ventricular contraction when the tricuspid and mitral (AV) valves are closing. The second heart sound ("dupp") occurs during ventricular relaxation when the pulmonic and aortic (SL) valves are closing.

## BLOOD FLOW THROUGH THE HEART

The right atrium receives blood low in oxygen and high in carbon dioxide from the superior and inferior vena cavae and the coronary sinus (Figure 1-5). Blood flows from the right atrium through the tricuspid valve into the right ventricle. When the right ventricle contracts, the tricuspid valve closes. The right ventricle expels the blood through the pulmonic valve into the pulmonary trunk. The pulmonary trunk divides into a right and left pulmonary artery, each of which carries blood to one lung (pulmonary circuit).

Blood flows through the pulmonary arteries to the lungs (where oxygen and carbon dioxide are exchanged in the pulmonary capillaries) and then to the pulmonary veins. The left atrium receives oxygenated blood from the lungs via the four pulmonary veins (two from the right lung and two from the left lung). Blood flows from the left atrium through the mitral (bicuspid) valve into the left

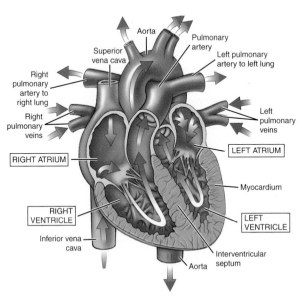

**Figure 1-5**   Blood flow through the heart.

ventricle. When the left ventricle contracts, the mitral valve closes. Blood leaves the left ventricle through the aortic valve to the aorta and its branches and is distributed throughout the body (systemic circuit). Blood from the tissues of the head, neck, and upper extremities is emptied into the superior vena cava. Blood from the lower body is emptied into the inferior vena cava. The superior and inferior vena cavae carry their blood into the right atrium.

## CARDIAC CYCLE

The cardiac cycle refers to a repetitive pumping process that includes all of the events associated with blood flow through the heart. The cycle has two phases for each heart chamber: systole and diastole. Systole is the period during which the chamber is contracting and blood is being ejected. Systole includes contraction of both atrial and ventricular muscle. Diastole is the period of relaxation during which the chambers are allowed to fill. Both the atria and ventricles have a diastolic phase. The myocardium receives its fresh supply of oxygenated blood during diastole. The cardiac cycle depends on the ability of the cardiac muscle to contract and on the condition of the heart's conduction system. The efficiency of the heart as a pump may be affected by abnormalities of the cardiac muscle, the valves, or the conduction system.

During the cardiac cycle, the pressure within each chamber of the heart rises in systole and falls in diastole. The heart's valves ensure that blood flows in the proper direction. Blood flows from one heart chamber to another if the pressure in the chamber is more than the pressure in the next. These pressure relationships depend on the careful timing of contractions. The heart's conduction system provides the necessary timing of events between atrial and ventricular systole.

## CORONARY CIRCULATION

### Coronary Arteries

In order to ensure that it has an adequate blood supply, the heart makes sure to provide itself with a fresh supply of oxygenated blood before supplying the rest of the body. This freshly oxygenated blood is supplied mainly by the branches of two vessels—the right and left coronary arteries. The right and left coronary arteries are the very first branches off the proximal aorta. The openings to these vessels are just beyond the cusps of the aortic SL valve. When the heart contracts, blood flow to the tissues of the heart is significantly reduced because the heart's blood vessels are compressed. Thus the coronary arteries fill when the ventricles are relaxed (diastole).

The main coronary arteries lie on the outer (epicardial) surface of the heart. They branch into progressively smaller vessels, eventually becoming arterioles, and then capillaries. Thus, the epicardium has a rich blood supply to draw from. Branches of the main coronary arteries penetrate into the heart's muscle mass and supply the subendocardium with blood. The diameter of these "feeder branches" (collateral circulation) is much narrower. The tissue supplied by these "feeder branches" gets enough blood and oxygen to survive, but they do not have much extra blood flow.

The three major coronary arteries include the left anterior descending (LAD), circumflex (CX), and right coronary arteries (RCA). The areas of the heart supplied by the three major coronary arteries are shown in Table 1-3.

### Right Coronary Artery

The right coronary artery (RCA) originates from the right side of the aorta. It travels along the groove between the right atrium and right ventricle. A branch of the RCA supplies the:

- Right atrium
- Right ventricle
- Inferior surface of the left ventricle in about 85% of individuals
- Posterior surface of the left ventricle in 85%
- Sinoatrial (SA) node in about 60%
- Atrioventricular (AV) node in 85% to 90%

### Left Coronary Artery

The left coronary artery (LCA) originates from the left side of the aorta. The first segment of the LCA is called the left main coronary artery. It is approximately the width of a soda straw and less than an inch long. The left main coronary artery supplies oxygenated blood to its two primary branches: the

| Table **1-3** | Coronary Arteries | |
|---|---|---|
| **Coronary Artery and Its Branches** | **Portion of Myocardium Supplied** | **Portion of Conduction System Supplied** |
| **RIGHT** | | |
| • Posterior descending<br>• Right marginal | • Right atrium<br>• Right ventricle<br>• Inferior surface of left ventricle (about 85%*)<br>• Posterior surface of left ventricle (about 85%*) | • SA node (about 60%*)<br>• AV node (85% to 90%*)<br>• Proximal portion of bundle of His<br>• Part of posterior-inferior fascicle of left bundle branch |
| **LEFT** | | |
| • Anterior descending | • Anterior surface of left ventricle<br>• Part of lateral surface of left ventricle<br>• Most of the interventricular septum | • Most of right bundle branch<br>• Anterior-superior fascicle of left bundle branch<br>• Part of posterior-inferior fascicle of left bundle branch |
| • Circumflex | • Left atrium<br><br>• Part of lateral surface of left ventricle<br>• Inferior surface of left ventricle (about 15%*)<br>• Posterior surface of left ventricle (15%*) | • SA node (about 40%*)<br>• AV node (10% to 15%*) |

*Of population

left anterior descending (LAD) (also called the *anterior interventricular*) artery and the left circumflex artery (LCx). These vessels are slightly smaller than the left main coronary artery.

The LAD can be seen on the outer (epicardial) surface on the front of the heart. It travels along the groove that lies between the right and left ventricles (anterior interventricular sulcus) toward the heart's apex. In more than 75% of patients, the LAD travels around the apex of the left ventricle and ends along the left ventricle's inferior surface. In the remaining patients, the LAD doesn't reach the inferior surface. Instead, it stops at or before the heart's apex. The major branches of the LAD are the septal and diagonal arteries. The septal branches of the LAD supply blood to the interventricular septum. The LAD supplies blood to:

- Anterior surface of left ventricle
- Part of lateral surface of left ventricle
- Most of the interventricular septum

The circumflex coronary artery circles around the left side of the heart. It is embedded in the epicardium on the back of the heart. The CX supplies blood to the:

- Left atrium
- Lateral surface of the left ventricle
- Inferior surface of the left ventricle in about 15% of individuals
- Posterior surface of the left ventricle in 15%
- SA node in about 40%
- AV node in 10% to 15%

## Coronary Veins

The coronary (cardiac) veins travel alongside the arteries. The coronary sinus is the largest vein that drains the heart. It lies in the groove that separates the atria from the ventricles. Blood that has passed through the myocardial capillaries is drained by branches of the cardiac veins that join the coronary sinus.

# HEART RATE

The heart is affected by both the sympathetic and parasympathetic divisions of the autonomic nervous system. The sympathetic division prepares the body to function under stress ("fight-or-flight" response). The parasympathetic division conserves and restores body resources ("feed-and-breed" or "rest and digest" response). A review of the autonomic nervous system can be found in Table 1-4.

## Baroreceptors and Chemoreceptors

Baroreceptors are specialized nerve tissue (sensors). They are found in the internal carotid arteries and the aortic arch. These sensory receptors detect changes in blood pressure. When they are stimulated, they cause a reflex response in either the sympathetic or the parasympathetic divisions of the autonomic nervous system. For example, if the blood pressure decreases, the body will attempt to compensate by:

- Constricting peripheral blood vessels
- Increasing heart rate (chronotropy)
- Increasing the force of myocardial contraction (inotropy)

| Chronotropic Effect | Inotropic Effect |
|---|---|
| • Refers to a change in heart rate | • Refers to a change in myocardial contractility |
| • A positive chronotropic effect refers to an increase in heart rate | • A positive inotropic effect results in an increase in myocardial contractility |
| • A negative chronotropic effect refers to a decrease in heart rate | • A negative inotropic effect results in a decrease in myocardial contractility |

These compensatory responses occur because of a response by the sympathetic division. This is called a *sympathetic or adrenergic response*. If the blood pressure increases, the body will decrease sympathetic stimulation and increase the response by the parasympathetic division. This is called a *parasympathetic or cholinergic response.*

Chemoreceptors in the internal carotid arteries and aortic arch detect changes in the concentration of hydrogen ions (pH), oxygen, and carbon dioxide in the blood. The response to these changes by the autonomic nervous system can be sympathetic or parasympathetic.

## Parasympathetic Stimulation

### Parasympathetic Receptor Sites

Parasympathetic (inhibitory) nerve fibers supply the SA node, atrial muscle, and the AV junction of the heart by means of the vagus nerves. Acetylcholine is a chemical messenger (neurotransmitter) that is released when parasympathetic nerves are stimulated. Acetylcholine binds to parasympathetic receptors. The two main types of parasympathetic receptors are nicotinic and muscarinic receptors. Nicotinic receptors are located in skeletal muscle. Muscarinic receptors are located in smooth muscle. Parasympathetic stimulation:

- Slows the rate of discharge of the SA node
- Slows conduction through the AV node
- Decreases the strength of atrial contraction
- Can cause a small decrease in the force of ventricular contraction

## Sympathetic Stimulation

Sympathetic (accelerator) nerves supply specific areas of the heart's electrical system, atrial muscle, and the ventricular myocardium. When sympathetic nerves are stimulated, norepinephrine is released. Remember: the job of the sympathetic division is to prepare the body for emergency or stressful situations. So, the release of norepinephrine results in some very predictable results:

- Increased force of contraction
- Increased heart rate
- Increased blood pressure

## Sympathetic Receptor Sites

Sympathetic (adrenergic) receptor sites are divided into alpha-receptors, beta-receptors, and dopaminergic receptors. Dopaminergic receptor sites are located in the coronary arteries and renal, mesenteric, and visceral blood vessels. Stimulation of dopaminergic receptor sites results in dilation.

| Table **1-4** | Review of the Autonomic Nervous System | |
|---|---|---|
| | Sympathetic Division | Parasympathetic Division |
| General effect | Fight or flight | Conserve resources ("Feed and breed" or "Rest and digest") |
| Primary neurotransmitter | Norepinephrine | Acetylcholine |
| **EFFECTS OF STIMULATION** | | |
| Abdominal blood vessels | Constriction (alpha-receptors) | No effect |
| Adrenal medulla | Increased secretion of epinephrine | No effect |
| Bronchioles | Dilation (beta-receptors) | Constriction |
| Blood vessels of skin | Constriction (alpha-receptors) | No effect |
| Blood vessels of skeletal muscle | Dilation (beta-receptors) | No effect |
| Cardiac muscle | Increased rate and strength of contraction (beta-receptors) | Decreased rate; decreased strength of atrial contraction, little effect on strength of ventricular contraction |
| Coronary blood vessels | Constriction (alpha-receptors) Dilation (beta-receptors) | Dilation |

# THE HEART AS A PUMP

## Venous Return

The heart functions as a pump to propel blood through the systemic and pulmonary circulations. As the heart chambers fill with blood, the heart muscle is stretched. The most important factor determining the amount of blood pumped out by the heart is the amount of blood flowing into it from the systemic circulation (venous return).

## Cardiac Output

Cardiac output is the amount of blood pumped into the aorta each minute by the heart. It is defined as the stroke volume (amount of blood ejected from a ventricle with each heartbeat) × the heart rate. In the average adult, normal cardiac output is between 4 and 8 L/min. The cardiac output at rest is about 5 L/min (stroke volume of 70 mL × a heart rate of 70 beats/min).

## Blood Pressure

The mechanical activity of the heart is reflected by the pulse and blood pressure. Blood pressure is the force exerted by the circulating blood volume on the walls of the arteries. Peripheral vascular resistance is the resistance to the flow of blood determined by blood vessel diameter and the tone of the vascular musculature. Blood pressure is equal to cardiac output × peripheral vascular resistance. Blood pressure is affected by any condition that increases peripheral resistance or cardiac output. Thus an increase in either cardiac output or peripheral resistance will result in an increase in blood pressure. Conversely, a decrease in either will result in a decrease in blood pressure.

### Stroke Volume
#### Preload
Stroke volume is determined by:

- The degree of ventricular filling when the heart is relaxed (preload)
- The pressure against which the ventricle must pump (afterload)
- The myocardium's contractile state (contracting or relaxing)

Preload is the force exerted on the walls of the ventricles at the end of diastole. The volume of blood returning to the heart influences preload. More blood returning to the right atrium increases preload. Less blood returning decreases preload.

According to the Starling's law of the heart, to a point, the greater the volume of blood in the heart during diastole, the more forceful the cardiac contraction, and the more blood the ventricle will pump (stroke volume). This is important so that the heart can adjust its pumping capacity in response to changes in venous return, such as during exercise. If, however, the ventricle is stretched beyond its physiologic limit, cardiac output may fall because of volume overload and overstretching of the muscle fibers.

### Afterload

Afterload is the pressure or resistance against which the ventricles must pump to eject blood. Afterload is influenced by:

- Arterial blood pressure
- The ability of the arteries to become stretched (arterial distensibility)
- Arterial resistance

The lower the resistance (lower afterload), the more easily blood can be ejected. Increased afterload (increased resistance) results in increased cardiac workload.

# Basic Electrophysiology

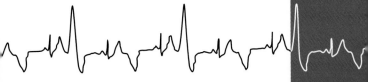

## TYPES OF CARDIAC CELLS

In general, cardiac cells have either a mechanical (contractile) or an electrical (pacemaker) function. Myocardial cells (working or mechanical cells) contain contractile filaments. When these cells are electrically stimulated, these filaments slide together, and the myocardial cell contracts. These myocardial cells form the thin muscular layer of the atrial walls and the thicker muscular layer of the ventricular walls (the myocardium). These cells do not normally generate electrical impulses on their own. They rely on pacemaker cells for this purpose.

Pacemaker cells are specialized cells of the heart's electrical system. They are responsible for spontaneously generating and conducting electrical impulses.

## CARDIAC ACTION POTENTIAL

Human body fluids contain electrolytes. Electrolytes are elements or compounds that break into charged particles (ions) when melted or dissolved in water or another solvent. The main electrolytes that affect the function of the heart are sodium (Na+), potassium (K+), calcium (Ca++), and chloride (Cl−). Body fluids that contain electrolytes conduct an electric current. Electrolytes move about in body fluids and carry a charge, just as electrons moving along a wire conduct current. The action potential is a five-phase cycle that reflects the difference in the concentration of these charged particles across the cell membrane at any given time.

## Polarization

In the body, cells spend a lot of time moving ions back and forth across their cell membranes. As a result, there is normally a slight difference in the concentrations of charged particles across the membranes of cells. Thus, there is potential energy (voltage) because of the imbalance of charged particles. This imbalance makes the cells excitable.

Cell membranes contain pores or channels through which specific electrolytes and other small, water-soluble molecules can cross the cell membrane from outside to inside (Figure 2-1).

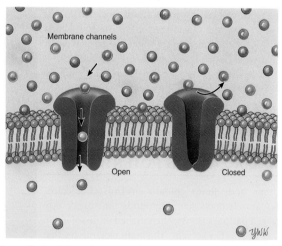

**Figure 2-1**    Cell membranes contain membrane channels. These channels are pores through which specific ions or other small, water-soluble molecules can cross the cell membrane from outside to inside.

When a cell is at rest, K+ leaks out of it. Large molecules such as proteins and phosphates remain inside the cell because they are too big to pass easily through the cell membrane. These large molecules carry a negative charge. This results in more negatively charged ions on the inside of the cell. When the inside of a cell is more negative than the outside it is polarized (Figure 2-2). The voltage (difference in electrical charges) across the cell membrane is the membrane potential. Electrolytes are quickly moved from one side of the cell membrane to the other by means of "pumps." These pumps require energy. The energy expended by the cells to move electrolytes across the cell membrane creates a flow of current. This flow of current is expressed in volts. Voltage can be measured and appears on an electrocardiogram (ECG) as spikes or waveforms. Thus an ECG is actually a sophisticated voltmeter.

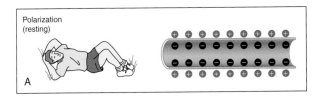

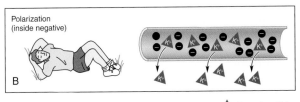

**Figure 2-2**  **A** and **B,** Polarization. When the inside of a cell is more negative than the outside it is said to be polarized.

## Depolarization

In order for a pacemaker cell to "fire" (produce an impulse), there must be a flow of electrolytes across the cell membrane. When a cell is stimulated, the cell membrane changes and becomes permeable to Na+ and K+. Na+ rushes into the cell through Na+ channels. This causes the inside of the cell to become more positive. A spike (waveform) is then recorded on the ECG. The stimulus that alters the electrical charges across the cell membrane may be electrical, mechanical, or chemical.

When opposite charges come together, energy is released. When the movement of electrolytes changes the electrical charge of the inside of the cell from negative to positive, an impulse is generated. The impulse causes channels to open in the next cell membrane and then the next. The movement of charged particles across a cell membrane causing the inside of the cell to become positive is called depolarization (Figure 2-3). Normally, an impulse begins in the pacemaker cells found in the sinoatrial (SA) node of the heart. A chain reaction occurs from cell to cell in the heart's electrical conduction system until all of the cells have been stimulated and depolarized. This chain reaction is called a wave of depolarization. The chain reaction is made possible because of the gap junctions that exist between the cells. Eventually, the impulse is spread from the pacemaker cells to the working myocardial cells. The working myocardial cells contract when they are stimulated. When the atria are stimulated, a P wave is recorded on the ECG. Thus the P wave represents atrial depolarization. When the ventricles are stimulated, a QRS complex is recorded on the ECG. Thus the QRS complex represents ventricular depolarization.

## Repolarization

After the cell depolarizes, it quickly begins to recover and restore its electrical charges to normal. The movement of charged particles across a cell membrane in which the inside of the cell is restored to its negative charge is called repolarization.

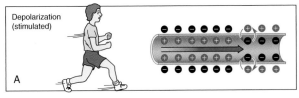

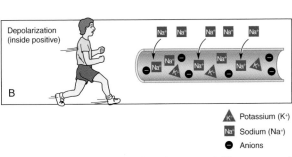

K⁺  Potassium (K⁺)

Na⁺  Sodium (Na⁺)

⬤  Anions

**Figure 2-3**  **A** and **B,** Depolarization is the movement of ions across a cell membrane causing the inside of the cell to become more positive.

The cell stops the flow of Na+ into the cell and allows K+ to leave it. Negatively charged particles are left inside the cell. Thus, the cell is returned to its resting state (Figure 2-4). This causes contractile proteins in the working myocardial cells to separate (relax). The cell can be stimulated again if another electrical impulse arrives at the cell membrane. Repolarization proceeds from the epicardium to the endocardium. On the ECG, the ST-segment and T wave represent ventricular repolarization.

## Phases of the Cardiac Action Potential

The action potential of a cardiac cell consists of five phases labeled 0 to 4. These phases reflect the rapid sequence of voltage changes that occur across the cell membrane during the electrical cardiac cycle. Phases 1, 2, and 3 have been referred to as *electrical systole*. Phase 4 has been referred to as *electrical*

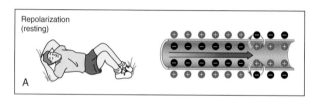

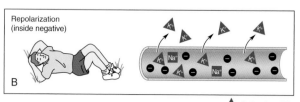

K — Potassium (K⁺)

Na — Sodium (Na⁺)

● — Anions

**Figure 2-4**   **A** and **B,** Repolarization is the movement of charged particles across a cell membrane in which the inside of the cell is restored to its negative charge.

*diastole.* The configuration of the action potential varies depending on the location, size, and function of the cardiac cell. Figure 2-5 shows the action potential of a normal ventricular muscle cell.

## PROPERTIES OF CARDIAC CELLS

The heart has pacemaker cells that can generate an electrical impulse without being stimulated by a nerve. The ability of cardiac pacemaker cells to create an electrical impulse without being stimulated from another source is called automaticity. Automaticity is a property of all cells of the heart. However, the heart's normal pacemaker usually prevents other areas of the heart from assuming this function.

Excitability (irritability) refers to the ability of cardiac muscle cells to respond to an outside stimulus. The stimulus may be from a chemical, mechanical, or electrical source.

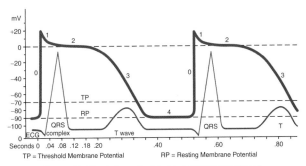

**Figure 2-5**   Action potential of a ventricular muscle cell.

Conductivity refers to the ability of a cardiac cell to receive an electrical impulse and conduct it to an adjoining cardiac cell. All cardiac cells possess this characteristic.

Contractility refers to the ability of myocardial cells to shorten in response to an impulse. This results in contraction. Normally, the heart contracts in response to an impulse that begins in the SA node.

## REFRACTORY PERIODS

Refractoriness is a term used to describe the period of recovery that cells need after being discharged before they are able to respond to a stimulus. In the heart, the refractory period is longer than the contraction itself.

### Absolute Refractory Period

During the absolute refractory period (also known as the effective refractory period), the cell will not respond to further stimulation. This means that the myocardial working cells cannot contract and the cells of the electrical conduction system cannot conduct an electrical impulse—no matter how strong the stimulus.

## Relative Refractory Period

During the relative refractory period (also known as the vulnerable period), some cardiac cells have repolarized to their threshold potential and can be stimulated to respond (depolarize) to a stronger than normal stimulus (Figure 2-6). This period corresponds with the downslope of the T wave on the ECG.

## Supernormal Period

After the relative refractory period is a supernormal period. A weaker than normal stimulus can cause cardiac cells to depolarize during this period. On the ECG, this corresponds with the end of the T wave. It is possible for dysrhythmias to develop during this period (see Figure 2-7).

## CONDUCTION SYSTEM

Figure 2-8 shows the heart's conduction system. A summary of the conduction system is shown in Table 2-1 (see page 30).

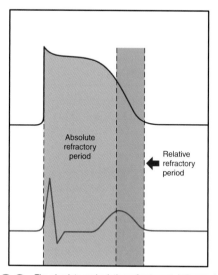

**Figure 2-6**    The absolute and relative refractory periods correlated with the action potential of a cardiac muscle cell and an ECG tracing.

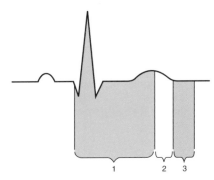

**Figure 2-7** (1) The absolute refractory period, (2) relative refractory period, and (3) the supernormal period.

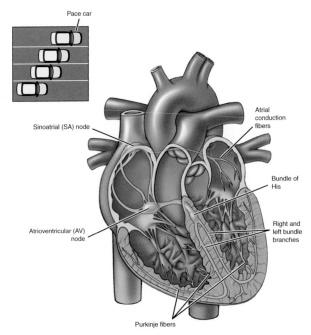

**Figure 2-8** The conduction system.

| Table **2-1** | Summary of the Conduction System | | |
|---|---|---|---|
| Structure | Location | Function | Intrinsic Pacemaker |
| SA node | Right atrial wall just inferior to opening of superior vena cava | Primary pace-maker; initiates impulse that is normally conducted throughout the left and right atria | 60-100 beats/min |
| AV node | Floor of the right atrium immediately behind the tricuspid valve and near the opening of the coronary sinus | Receives impulse from SA node and delays relay of the impulse to the bundle of His, allowing time for the atria to empty their contents into the ventricles before the onset of ventricular contraction. | |
| Bundle of His | Superior portion of interventricular septum | Receives impulse from AV node and relays it to right and left bundle branches | 40-60 beats/min |
| Right and left bundle branches | Interventricular septum | Receives impulse from bundle of His and relays it to Purkinje fibers | |
| Purkinje fibers | Ventricular myocardium | Receives impulse from bundle branches and relays it to ventricular myocardium | 20-40 beats/min |

## Electrocardiogram

ECG monitoring may be used to:

- Monitor a patient's heart rate
- Evaluate the effects of disease or injury on heart function
- Evaluate pacemaker function
- Evaluate the response to medications (e.g., antiarrhythmics)
- Obtain a baseline recording before, during, and after a medical procedure

The ECG *can* provide information about:

- The orientation of the heart in the chest
- Conduction disturbances
- Electrical effects of medications and electrolytes
- The mass of cardiac muscle
- The presence of ischemic damage

The ECG does *not* provide information about the mechanical (contractile) condition of the myocardium. To evaluate the effectiveness of the heart's mechanical activity, you must assess the patient's pulse and blood pressure.

## Electrodes

It is important to define three terms: Electrode, cable, and lead.

- **Electrode** refers to the paper, plastic, or metal device that contains conductive media and is applied to the patient's skin. Electrodes are applied at specific locations on the patient's chest wall and extremities to view the heart's electrical activity from different angles and planes.
- **Cable** refers to the wire that attaches to the electrode and conducts current back to the cardiac monitor. One end of a monitoring cable is attached to the electrode and the other end to an ECG machine.
- **Lead** is used in two ways. The term lead refers to the actual tracing obtained and the position of the electrode. For example, the term "$V_1$ position" represents its proper location on the chest wall, while "lead $V_1$" refers to the tracing obtained from that position.

## Leads

A lead is a record (tracing) of electrical activity between two electrodes. Each lead records the *average* current flow at a specific time in a portion of the heart. Leads allow viewing the heart's electrical activity in two different planes: frontal (coronal) and horizontal (transverse). Frontal plane leads view the heart from the front of the body. Horizontal plane leads view the heart as if the body were sliced in half horizontally. A 12-lead ECG provides views of the heart in both the frontal and horizontal planes and views the surfaces of the left ventricle from 12 different angles.

There are three types of leads: standard limb leads, augmented limb leads, and chest (precordial) leads. Each lead has a negative (−) and positive (+) electrode (pole). Moving the lead selector on the ECG machine allows the electrodes to be made positive or negative.

When electrical activity is not detected, a straight line is recorded. This line is called the baseline or isoelectric line. A waveform (deflection) is movement away from the baseline in a positive (upward) or negative (downward) direction. If the wave of depolarization (electrical impulse) moves toward the positive electrode, the waveform recorded on ECG graph paper will be upright (positive deflection). If the wave of depolarization moves toward the negative electrode, the waveform recorded will be inverted (downward or negative deflection). A biphasic (partly positive, partly negative) waveform or a straight line is recorded when the wave of depolarization moves perpendicularly to the positive electrode.

### Frontal Plane Leads

Frontal plane leads view the heart from the front of the body as if it were flat (Figure 2-9). Directions in the frontal plane are superior, inferior, right, and left. Six leads view the heart in the frontal plane: three bipolar leads and three unipolar leads.

A bipolar lead is an ECG lead that has a positive and negative electrode. Each lead records the difference in electrical potential

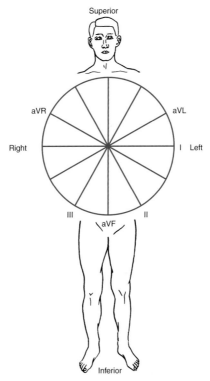

**Figure 2-9**  Frontal plane leads.

between two selected electrodes. Leads I, II, and III are called *standard limb leads* or *bipolar leads*.

A lead that consists of a single positive electrode and a reference point is called a unipolar lead. These leads are also called *unipolar limb leads* or *augmented limb leads*. The reference point (with zero electrical potential) lies in the center of the heart's electrical field (left of the interventricular septum and below the AV junction).

Leads aVR, aVL, and aVF are augmented limb leads (Figure 2-10). The electrical potential produced by the augmented leads is normally relatively small. The ECG machine augments (magnifies) the amplitude of the electrical potentials detected at each extremity by about 50% over those recorded at the bipolar leads.

### Horizontal Plane Leads

Horizontal plane leads view the heart as if the body were sliced in half horizontally. Directions in the horizontal plane are anterior, posterior, right, and left. Six chest (precordial or "V") leads view the heart in the horizontal plane (Figure 2-11). This allows a view of the front and left side of the heart. The chest leads are identified as $V_1$, $V_2$, $V_3$, $V_4$, $V_5$, and $V_6$. Each electrode placed in a "V" position is a positive electrode. The negative electrode is found at the electrical center of the heart. Thus the chest leads are also unipolar leads.

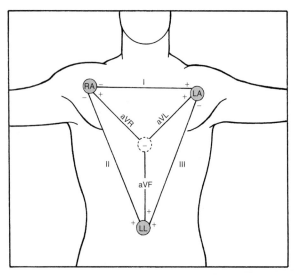

**Figure 2-10**    View of the standard limb leads and augmented leads.

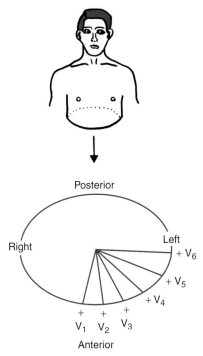

**Figure 2-11** Horizontal plane leads.

## Standard Limb Leads

Leads I, II, and III make up the standard limb leads. If an electrode is placed on the right arm, left arm, and left leg, three leads are formed. Since each of these three leads has a distinct negative pole and a distinct positive pole, they are considered bipolar. The positive electrode is located at the left wrist in lead I, while leads II and III both have their positive electrode located at the left foot. The difference in electrical potential between the positive pole and its corresponding negative pole is measured by each lead. A summary of the standard limb leads can be found in Table 2-2.

| Table **2-2** | Summary of Standard Limb Leads | | |
| Lead | Positive Electrode | Negative Electrode | Heart Surface Viewed |
| --- | --- | --- | --- |
| I | Left arm | Right arm | Lateral |
| II | Left leg | Right arm | Inferior |
| III | Left leg | Left arm | Inferior |

## Augmented Limb Leads

Leads aVR, aVL, and aVF are augmented limb leads. The electrical potential produced by the augmented leads is normally relatively small. The ECG machine augments (magnifies) the amplitude of the electrical potentials detected at each extremity by approximately 50% over those recorded at the bipolar leads. The "a" in aVR, aVL, and aVF refers to augmented. The "V" refers to voltage. The "R" refers to right arm, the "L" to left arm, and the "F" to left foot (leg). The position of the positive electrode corresponds to the last letter in each of these leads. The positive electrode in aVR is located on the right arm, aVL has a positive electrode at the left arm, and aVF has a positive electrode positioned on the left leg.

While leads aVR, aVL, and aVF have a distinct positive pole, they do not have a distinct negative pole. Since they have only one true pole, they are referred to as unipolar leads. In place of a single negative pole these leads have multiple negative poles, creating a negative field (central terminal), of which the heart is at the center. Theoretically, this makes the heart the negative electrode. A summary of augmented leads can be found in Table 2-3.

| Table **2-3** | Summary of Augmented Leads | |
| Lead | Positive Electrode | Heart Surface Viewed |
| --- | --- | --- |
| aVR | Right arm | None |
| aVL | Left arm | Lateral |
| aVF | Left leg | Inferior |

## Chest Leads

The six chest leads are unipolar leads that view the heart in the horizontal plane. The chest leads are identified as $V_1$, $V_2$, $V_3$, $V_4$, $V_5$, and $V_6$. Each electrode placed in a V position is a positive electrode. Because the chest leads are unipolar, the positive electrode for each lead is placed at a specific location on the chest. The heart is the theoretical negative electrode. A summary of the chest leads can be found in Table 2-4.

| Table **2-4** | Summary of Chest Leads | |
|---|---|---|
| Lead | Positive Electrode Position | Heart Surface Viewed |
| $V_1$ | Right side of sternum, 4th intercostal space | Septum |
| $V_2$ | Left side of sternum, 4th intercostal space | Septum |
| $V_3$ | Midway between $V_2$ and $V_4$ | Anterior |
| $V_4$ | Left midclavicular line, 5th intercostal space | Anterior |
| $V_5$ | Left anterior axillary line at same level as $V_4$ | Lateral |
| $V_6$ | Left midaxillary line at same level as $V_4$ | Lateral |

### Right Chest Leads

Other chest leads that are not part of a standard 12-lead ECG may be used to view specific surfaces of the heart. When a right ventricular myocardial infarction is suspected, right chest leads are used. Placement of right chest leads is identical to placement of the standard chest leads except it is done on the right side of the chest. If time does not permit obtaining all of the right chest leads, the lead of choice is $V_4R$. The right chest leads and their placement are shown in Figure 2-12.

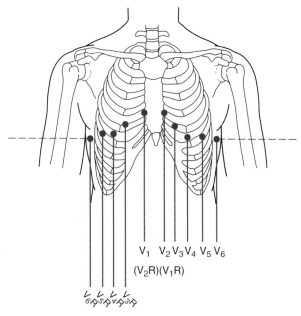

$V_1$   $V_2$ $V_3$ $V_4$   $V_5$ $V_6$

$(V_2R)(V_1R)$

**Figure 2-12**   Anatomic placement of the left and right chest leads.

### Posterior Chest Leads

On a standard 12-lead ECG, no leads look directly at the posterior surface of the heart. Additional chest leads may be used for this purpose. These leads are placed further left and toward the back. All of the leads are placed on the same horizontal line as $V_4$ to $V_6$. Lead $V_7$ is placed at the posterior axillary line. Lead $V_8$ is placed at the angle of the scapula (posterior scapular line) and lead $V_9$ is placed over the left border of spine (Figure 2-13).

## ECG PAPER

Remember that the ECG is a graphical representation of the heart's electrical activity. When you place electrodes on the patient's body and connect them to an ECG, the machine

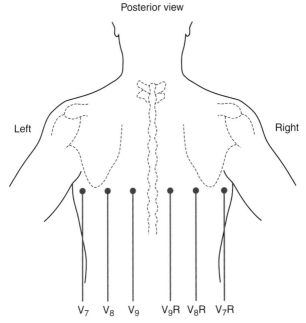

**Figure 2-13**  Posterior chest lead placement.

records the voltage (potential difference) between the electrodes. The needle (or pen) of the ECG moves a specific distance depending on the voltage measured. This recording is made on ECG paper.

ECG paper is graph paper made up of small and large boxes measured in millimeters. The smallest boxes are 1 mm wide and 1 mm high. The horizontal axis of the paper corresponds with *time*. Time is used to measure the interval between or duration of specific cardiac events. Time is stated in seconds.

The rate at which ECG paper goes through the printer is adjustable. Standard paper speed is 25 mm/sec. ECG paper normally records at a constant speed of 25 mm/sec. Thus, each horizontal 1-mm box represents 0.04 second (25 mm/sec × 0.04 sec = 1 mm). Look closely at the boxes in Figure 2-14. You can see that the lines after every five small boxes on the paper are heavier. The heavier lines indicate one large box. Because each large box is the width of five small boxes, a large box represents 0.20 second.

The vertical axis of the ECG paper measures the *voltage* or *amplitude* of a waveform. Voltage is measured in millivolts (mV). Voltage may be a positive or negative value. Amplitude is measured in millimeters (mm). The ECG machine's sensitivity must be calibrated so that a 1-mV electrical signal will produce a deflection measuring exactly 10 mm tall. When properly calibrated, a small box is 1 mm high (0.1 mV), and a large box (equal to five small boxes) is 5 mm high (0.5 mV). Clinically, the height of a waveform is usually stated in millimeters, not millivolts.

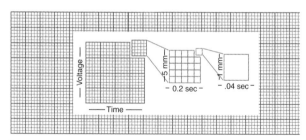

**Figure 2-14**    The horizontal axis represents time. The vertical axis represents amplitude or voltage.

## WAVEFORMS

A waveform is movement away from the baseline in either a positive (upward) or negative (downward) direction. Waveforms are named alphabetically, beginning with P, QRS, T, and U. A waveform that is partly positive and partly negative is biphasic. A waveform that rests on the baseline is isoelectric.

## P Wave

Remember that an impulse that begins in the SA node is not recorded on the ECG. However, the spread of that impulse throughout the atria (atrial depolarization) is observed. The first waveform in the cardiac cycle is the *P wave*. The first half of the P wave is recorded when the electrical impulse that originated in the SA node stimulates the right atrium and reaches the AV node. The downslope of the P wave reflects stimulation of the left atrium. Thus the P wave represents atrial depolarization and the spread of the electrical impulse throughout the right and left atria.

The atria contract a fraction of a second after the P wave begins. The atria begin to repolarize at the same time as the ventricles depolarize. A waveform representing atrial repolarization is usually not seen on the ECG because it is small and buried in the QRS complex.

The beginning of the P wave is recognized as the first abrupt or gradual deviation from the baseline; its end is the point at which the waveform returns to the baseline (Figure 2-15).

### Normal Characteristics of the P Wave
- Smooth and rounded
- No more than 2.5 mm in height
- No more than 0.11 second in duration
- Positive in leads I, II, aVF, and $V_2$ through $V_6$

## QRS Complex

A complex consists of several waveforms. The QRS complex consists of the Q wave, R wave, and S wave. It represents the spread of the electrical impulse through the ventricles (ventricular depolarization). Normally, depolarization triggers contraction of ventricular tissue. Thus, shortly after the QRS complex begins, the ventricles contract (Figure 2-16). The QRS complex is significantly larger than the P wave because depolarization of the ventricles involves a considerably greater muscle mass than depolarization of the atria. A QRS complex normally follows each P wave. One or even two of the three waveforms that make up the QRS complex may not always be present.

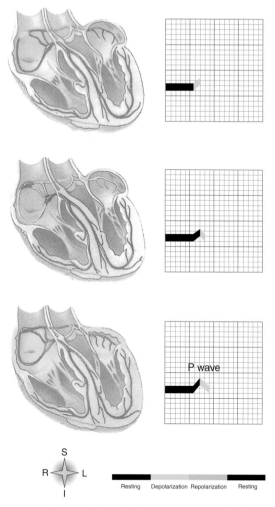

**Figure 2-15** The beginning of the P wave is recognized as the first abrupt or gradual deviation from the baseline. Its end is the point at which the waveform returns to the baseline.

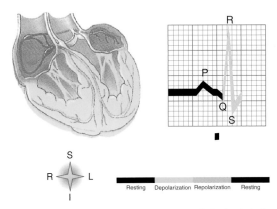

**Figure 2-16** The QRS complex represents ventricular depolarization.

The QRS duration is a measurement of the time required for ventricular depolarization. The width of a QRS complex is most accurately determined when it is viewed and measured in more than one lead. The measurement should be taken from the QRS complex with the longest duration and clearest onset and end. The beginning of the QRS complex is measured from the point where the first wave of the complex begins to deviate from the baseline. The point at which the last wave of the complex begins to level out or distinctly change direction at, above, or below the baseline marks the end of the QRS complex. In adults, the normal duration of the QRS complex varies between 0.06 and 0.10 second. If an electrical impulse does not follow the normal ventricular conduction pathway, it will take longer to depolarize the myocardium. This delay in conduction through the ventricle produces a wider QRS complex.

## Normal Characteristics of the QRS Complex

- Normal duration of the QRS complex in an adult varies between 0.06 and 0.10 second
- A normal Q wave is less than 0.04 second in duration and less than one third of the amplitude of the R wave in that lead

## T Wave

Ventricular repolarization is represented on the ECG by the T wave (Figure 2-17). The normal T wave is slightly asymmetric: the peak of the waveform is closer to its end than to the beginning, and the first half has a more gradual slope than the second half. The beginning of the T wave is identified as the point where the slope of the ST-segment appears to become abruptly or gradually steeper. The T wave ends when it returns to the baseline.

### Normal Characteristics of the T Wave
- Slightly asymmetric
- T waves are not normally more than 5 mm in height in any limb lead or 10 mm in any chest lead; T waves are not normally less than 0.5 mm in height in leads I and II

### U Wave

A U wave is a small waveform that, when seen, follows the T wave. The mechanism of the U wave is not definitely known. One theory suggests that it represents repolarization of the Purkinje fibers. Normal U waves are small, round, and less than 1.5 mm in amplitude. U waves are most easily seen when the heart rate is slow and

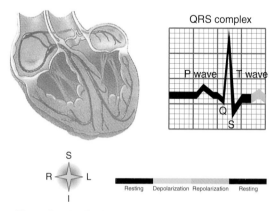

**Figure 2-17**   The T wave represents ventricular repolarization.

are difficult to identify when the rate exceeds 90 beats/min. When seen, they are normally tallest in leads $V_2$ and $V_3$. U waves usually appear in the same direction as the T wave that precedes it.

### Characteristics of the U Wave
- Rounded and symmetric
- Usually less than 1.5 mm in height and smaller than that of the preceding T wave
- In general, a U wave more than 1.5 mm in height in any lead is considered abnormal

## SEGMENTS

A segment is a line between waveforms. It is named by the waveform that precedes or follows it.

### PR-Segment

The PR-segment is the horizontal line between the end of the P wave and the beginning of the QRS complex (Figure 2-18). It represents activation of the AV node, the bundle of His, the bundle branches, and the Purkinje fibers.

### ST-segment

The portion of the ECG tracing between the QRS complex and the T wave is the ST-segment. The ST-segment represents the early part of repolarization of the right and left ventricles. The

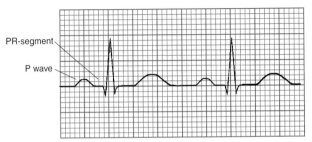

**Figure 2-18**  The PR-segment.

normal ST-segment begins at the isoelectric line, extends from the end of the S wave, and curves gradually upward to the beginning of the T wave.

The point where the QRS complex and the ST-segment meet is called the *junction* or *J-point*. Various conditions may cause displacement of the ST-segment from the isoelectric line in either a positive or negative direction. Myocardial ischemia, injury, and infarction are among the causes of ST-segment deviation.

## Normal Characteristics of the ST-segment

- Begins with the end of the QRS complex and ends with the onset of the T wave
- In the limb leads, the normal ST-segment is isoelectric (flat) but may normally be slightly elevated or depressed (usually by less than 1 mm)
- In the chest leads, ST-segment deviation may vary from −0.5 to +2 mm

## TP-segment

The TP-segment is the portion of the ECG tracing between the end of the T wave and the beginning of the following P wave (Figure 2-19). When the heart rate is within normal limits, the TP-segment is usually isoelectric. With rapid heart rates, the TP-segment is often unrecognizable because the P wave encroaches on the preceding T wave.

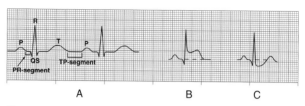

A          B          C

**Figure 2-19    A-C,** The TP-segment. **A,** The PR- and TP-segments are used as the baseline from which to determine the presence of ST-segment elevation or depression. **B,** ST-segment elevation. **C,** ST-segment depression.

## INTERVALS

### PR Interval

An interval is a waveform and a segment. The P wave plus the PR-segment equals the PR interval (PRI). The PR interval is measured from the point where the P wave leaves the baseline to the beginning of the QRS complex. The P wave reflects depolarization of the right and left atria. The PR-segment represents the spread of the impulse through the AV node, bundle of His, right and left bundle branches, and the Purkinje fibers. The PRI changes with heart rate but normally measures 0.12 to 0.20 second in adults. As the heart rate increases, the duration of the PR interval shortens. A conduction problem above the level of the bundle branches will largely affect the P wave and PR interval.

#### Normal Characteristics of the PR Interval
- Normally measures 0.12 to 0.20 second in adults; may be shorter in children and longer in older persons
- Normally shortens as heart rate increases

### QT Interval

The QT interval represents total ventricular activity—the time from ventricular depolarization (activation) to repolarization (recovery). The QT interval is measured from the beginning of the QRS complex to the end of the T wave. In the absence of a Q wave, the QT interval is measured from the beginning of the R wave to the end of the T wave. The duration of the QT interval varies according to age, gender, and heart rate.

### R-R and P-P Intervals

The R-to-R (R-R) and P-to-P (P-P) intervals are used to determine the rate and regularity of a cardiac rhythm. To evaluate the regularity of the ventricular rhythm on a rhythm strip, the interval between two consecutive R-R waves is measured. The distance between succeeding R-R intervals is measured and compared. If the ventricular rhythm is regular, the R-R intervals will measure the same.

To evaluate the regularity of the atrial rhythm, the same procedure is used but the interval between two consecutive P-P waves is measured and compared to succeeding P-P intervals.

## ANALYZING A RHYTHM STRIP

It is essential to develop a systematic approach to rhythm analysis and consistently apply it when analyzing a rhythm strip. If you do not develop such an approach, you are more likely to miss something important. Begin analyzing the rhythm strip from left to right.

### Assess Rhythm/Regularity

The term rhythm is used to indicate the site of origin of an electrical impulse (e.g., sinus rhythm, junctional rhythm) and to describe the regularity or irregularity of waveforms.

The waveforms on an ECG strip are evaluated for regularity by measuring the distance between the P waves and QRS complexes. If the rhythm is regular, the R-R intervals (or P-P intervals, if assessing atrial rhythm) are the same. Generally, a variation of plus or minus 10% is acceptable. For example, if there are 10 small boxes in an R-R interval, an R wave could be "off" by 1 small box and still be considered regular.

Various terms may be used to describe an irregular rhythm, which may be normal, fast, or slow. If the variation between the shortest and longest R-R intervals (or P-P intervals) is less than four small boxes (0.16 sec), the rhythm is termed essentially regular. For example, the underlying rhythm may be regular but the pattern may be periodically interrupted by ectopic beats that arise from a part of the heart other than the SA node.

If the shortest and longest R-R intervals vary by more than 0.16 second, the rhythm is considered irregular. A regularly irregular rhythm is one in which the R-R intervals are not the same, the shortest and longest R-R intervals vary by more than 0.16 second, and there is a repeating pattern of irregularity. A regularly irregular rhythm may be due to grouped beating (a repeating pattern of irregularity). An irregularly irregular rhythm is one in which the R-R intervals are not the same, there is no repeating pattern of irregularity, and the shortest and longest R-R intervals vary by more than 0.16 second. An irregularly irregular rhythm may also be called a grossly or totally irregular rhythm.

## Assess the Rate

There are several methods used for calculating heart rate (Figure 2-20). A discussion of each method follows.

### Method 1: Six-Second Method

Most ECG paper is printed with 1-second or 3-second markers on the top or bottom of the paper. On ECG paper, 5 large boxes = 1 second, 15 large boxes = 3 seconds, and 30 large boxes = 6 seconds. To determine the ventricular rate, count the number of complete QRS complexes within a period of 6 seconds and multiply that number by 10 to find the number of complexes in 1 minute. This method may be used for regular and irregular rhythms. This is the simplest, quickest, and most commonly used method of rate measurement, but it also is the most inaccurate.

### Method 2: Large Boxes

To determine the ventricular rate, count the number of large boxes between the R-R interval and divide into 300. To determine the atrial rate, count the number of large boxes between

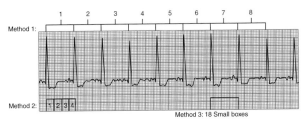

**Figure 2-20** Calculating heart rate. Method 1: Number of R-R intervals in 6 seconds × 10 (e.g., 8 × 10 = 80 beats/min). Method 2: Number of large boxes between QRS complexes divided into 300 (e.g., 300/4 = 75 beats/min). Method 3: Number of small boxes between QRS complexes divided into 1500 (e.g., 1500/18 = 84 beats/min).

the P-P interval and divide into 300 (Table 2-5). This method is best used if the rhythm is regular; however, it may be used if the rhythm is irregular and a rate range (slowest [longest R-R interval] and fastest [shortest R-R interval] rate) is given.

A variation of the large box method is called the sequence method. To determine ventricular rate, select an R wave that falls on a dark vertical line. Number the next six consecutive dark vertical lines as follows: 300, 150, 100, 75, 60, and 50 (Figure 2-21). Note where the next R wave falls in relation to the six dark vertical lines already marked. This is the heart rate.

### Method 3: Small Boxes
Each 1-mm box on the graph paper represents 0.04 second. A total of 1500 boxes represents 1 minute (60 sec/min divided by 0.04 sec/box = 1500 boxes/min). To calculate the ventricular rate, count the number of small boxes between the R-R interval and divide into 1500. To determine the atrial rate, count the number of small boxes between the P-P interval and divide into 1500. This method is time consuming but accurate. If the rhythm is irregular, a rate range should be given.

### Identify and Examine P Waves
To locate P waves, look to the left of each QRS complex. Normally, one P wave precedes each QRS complex, they occur regularly, and look similar in size, shape, and position. If no

| Table **2-5** | Heart Rate Determination Based on the Number of Large Boxes | | |
|---|---|---|---|
| Number of Large Boxes | Heart Rate (beats/min) | Number of Large Boxes | Heart Rate (beats/min) |
| 1 | 300 | 6 | 50 |
| 2 | 150 | 7 | 43 |
| 3 | 100 | 8 | 38 |
| 4 | 75 | 9 | 33 |
| 5 | 60 | 10 | 30 |

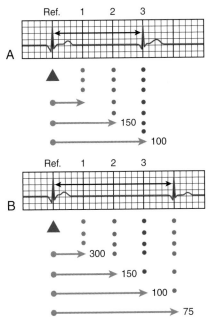

**Figure 2-21** **A** and **B,** Determining heart rate—sequence method. To measure the ventricular rate, find a QRS complex that falls on a heavy dark line. Count 300, 150, 100, 75, 60, and 50 until a second QRS complex occurs. This will be the heart rate. **A,** Heart rate = 100. **B,** Heart rate = 75.

P wave is present, the rhythm originated in the AV junction or the ventricles. If one P wave is present before each QRS and the QRS is *narrow* consider the following:

- Is the P wave positive? If so, the rhythm probably began in the SA node.
- Is the P wave negative or absent? If so, and the QRS complexes occur regularly, the rhythm probably started in the AV junction.

## Assess Intervals (Evaluate Conduction)

### PR Interval

Measure the PR interval. The PR interval is measured from the point where the P wave leaves the baseline to the beginning of the QRS complex. The normal PR interval is 0.12 to 0.20 second. If the PR intervals are the same, they are said to be constant. If the PR intervals are different, is there a pattern? In some dysrhythmias, the duration of the PR interval will increase until a P wave appears with no QRS after it. This is referred to as "lengthening" of the PR interval. PR intervals that vary in duration and have no pattern are said to be "variable."

### QRS Duration

Identify the QRS complexes and measure their duration. The beginning of the QRS is measured from the point where the first wave of the complex begins to deviate from the baseline. The point at which the last wave of the complex begins to level out at, above, or below the baseline marks the end of the QRS complex. The QRS is considered narrow (normal) if it measures 0.10 second or less and wide if it measures more than 0.10 second.

### QT Interval

Measure the QT interval in the leads that show the largest amplitude T waves. The QT interval is measured from the beginning of the QRS complex to the end of the T wave. If there is no Q wave, measure the QT interval from the beginning of the R wave to the end of the T wave. If the measured QT interval is less than half the R-R interval, it is probably normal. This method of QT interval measurement works well as a general guideline until the ventricular rate exceeds 100 beats/min.

## Evaluate the Overall Appearance of the Rhythm

### ST-segment

Determine the presence of ST-segment elevation or depression. The TP- and PR-segments are used as the baseline from which to evaluate the degree of displacement of the ST-segment from the isoelectric line. The ST-segment is considered elevated if the segment is deviated above the baseline and is considered depressed if the segment deviates below it.

### T Wave

Evaluate the T waves. Are the T waves upright and of normal height? The T wave following an abnormal QRS complex is usually opposite in direction of the QRS. Negative T waves suggest myocardial ischemia. Tall, pointed (peaked) T waves are commonly seen in hyperkalemia.

## Interpret the Rhythm and Evaluate Its Clinical Significance

Interpret the rhythm, specifying the site of origin (pacemaker site) of the rhythm (sinus), the mechanism (bradycardia), and the ventricular rate. For example, "Sinus bradycardia at 38 beats/min." Evaluate the patient's clinical presentation to determine how he or she is tolerating the rate and rhythm.

# Sinus Mechanisms

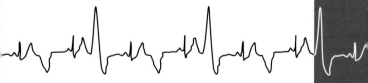

The normal heartbeat is the result of an electrical impulse that starts in the sinoatrial (SA) node. Normally, pacemaker cells within the SA node spontaneously depolarize more rapidly than other cardiac cells. As a result, the SA node usually dominates other areas that may be depolarizing at a slightly slower rate. The impulse is sent to cells at the outside edge of the SA node and then to the myocardial cells of the surrounding atrium.

A rhythm that begins in the SA node has:

- A positive (upright) P wave before each QRS complex
- P waves that look alike
- A constant PR interval
- A regular atrial and ventricular rhythm (usually)

## SINUS RHYTHM

Sinus rhythm is the name given to a normal heart rhythm. Sinus rhythm reflects normal electrical activity (i.e., the rhythm starts in the SA node and then heads down the normal conduction pathway through the atria, AV junction, bundle branches, and ventricles). In adults and adolescents, the SA node normally fires at a regular rate of 60 to 100 beats/min. An example of a sinus rhythm is shown in Figure 3-1. A summary of the ECG characteristics of a sinus rhythm are shown in Table 3-1.

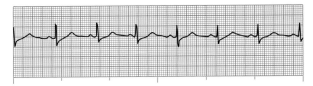

**Figure 3-1**   Sinus rhythm at 75 beats/min, ST-segment depression.

| Table **3-1** | Characteristics of Sinus Rhythm |
| --- | --- |
| Rate | 60-100 beats/min |
| Rhythm | P-P interval regular, R-R interval regular |
| P waves | Positive (upright) in lead II, one precedes each QRS complex, P waves look alike |
| PR interval | 0.12-0.20 sec and constant from beat to beat |
| QRS duration | 0.10 sec or less unless an intraventricular conduction delay exists |

## SINUS BRADYCARDIA

If the SA node fires at a rate slower than normal for the patient's age, the rhythm is called sinus bradycardia. In adults and adolescents, a sinus bradycardia has a heart rate of less than 60 beats/min. The term *severe sinus bradycardia* is sometimes used to describe a sinus bradycardia with a rate of less than 40 beats/min. An example of sinus bradycardia is shown in Figure 3-2. The ECG characteristics of sinus bradycardia are shown in Table 3-2.

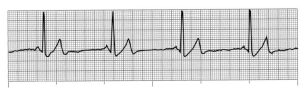

**Figure 3-2**   Sinus bradycardia at 46 beats/min, ST-segment depression.

| Table **3-2** | Characteristics of Sinus Bradycardia |
|---|---|
| Rate | Less than 60 beats/min |
| Rhythm | P-P interval regular, R-R interval regular |
| P waves | Positive (upright) in lead II, one precedes each QRS complex, P waves look alike |
| PR interval | 0.12-0.20 sec and constant from beat to beat |
| QRS duration | 0.10 sec or less unless an intraventricular conduction delay exists |

## SINUS TACHYCARDIA

If the SA node fires at a rate faster than normal for the patient's age, the rhythm is called sinus tachycardia. Sinus tachycardia begins and ends gradually. An example of sinus tachycardia is shown in Figure 3-3. The ECG characteristics of sinus tachycardia are shown in Table 3-3.

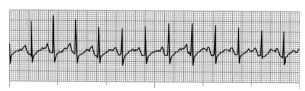

**Figure 3-3**    Sinus tachycardia at 125 beats/min, ST-segment depression.

| Table **3-3** | Characteristics of Sinus Tachycardia |
|---|---|
| Rate | 101-180 beats/min |
| Rhythm | P-P interval regular, R-R interval regular |
| P waves | Positive (upright) in lead II, one precedes each QRS complex, P waves look alike |
| | At very fast rates it may be hard to tell the difference between a P wave from a T wave |
| PR interval | 0.12-0.20 sec (may shorten with faster rates) and constant from beat to beat |
| QRS duration | 0.10 sec or less unless an intraventricular conduction delay exists |

# SINUS ARRHYTHMIA

When the SA node fires irregularly, the resulting rhythm is called sinus arrhythmia. Sinus arrhythmia that is associated with the phases of respiration and changes in intrathoracic pressure is called *respiratory sinus arrhythmia*. Sinus arrhythmia that is not related to the respiratory cycle is called *nonrespiratory sinus arrhythmia*. An example of sinus arrhythmia is shown in Figure 3-4. The characteristics of sinus arrhythmia are shown in Table 3-4.

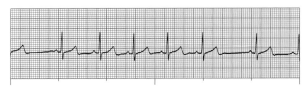

**Figure 3-4**    Sinus arrhythmia at 54 to 88 beats/min.

| Table 3-4 | Characteristics of Sinus Arrhythmia |
|---|---|
| Rate | Usually 60-100 beats/min, but may be slower or faster |
| Rhythm | Irregular, phasic with respiration; heart rate increases gradually during inspiration (R-R intervals shorten) and decreases with expiration (R-R intervals lengthen) |
| P waves | Positive (upright) in lead II, one precedes each QRS complex, P waves look alike |
| PR interval | 0.12-0.20 sec and constant from beat to beat |
| QRS duration | 0.10 sec or less unless an intraventricular conduction delay exists |

# SINOATRIAL (SA) BLOCK

In sinoatrial (SA) block, the pacemaker cells within the SA node initiate an impulse but it is blocked as it exits the SA node. This is thought to occur because of failure of the transitional cells in the SA node to conduct the impulse from the pacemaker cells to the surrounding atrium. An example of SA block is shown in Figure 3-5. The ECG characteristics of SA block are shown in Table 3-5.

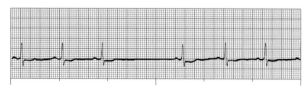

**Figure 3-5**  Sinus rhythm at a rate of 36 to 71 beats/min with an episode of sinoatrial (SA) block.

| Table **3-5** | Characteristics of Sinoatrial (SA) Block |
| --- | --- |
| Rate | Usually normal but varies because of the pause |
| Rhythm | Irregular due to the pause(s) caused by the SA block—the pause is the same as (or an exact multiple of) the distance between two other P-P intervals |
| P waves | Positive (upright) in lead II, P waves look alike. When present, one precedes each QRS complex. |
| P-R interval | 0.12-0.20 sec and constant from beat to beat |
| QRS duration | 0.10 sec or less unless an intraventricular conduction delay exists |

## SINUS ARREST

In sinus arrest, the pacemaker cells of the SA node fail to initiate an electrical impulse for one or more beats. When the SA node fails to initiate an impulse, an escape pacemaker site (the AV junction or ventricles) should assume responsibility for pacing the heart. If they do not, you will see absent PQRST complexes on the ECG. An example of sinus arrest is shown in Figure 3-6. The ECG characteristics of sinus arrest are shown in Table 3-6.

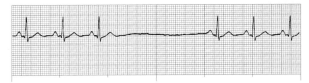

**Figure 3-6**    Sinus rhythm at a rate of 24 to 81 beats/min with an episode of sinus arrest.

| Table 3-6 | Characteristics of Sinus Arrest |
|---|---|
| Rate | Usually normal but varies because of the pause |
| Rhythm | Irregular—the pause is of undetermined length (more than one PQRST complex is missing) and is not the same distance as other P-P intervals |
| P waves | Positive (upright) in lead II, P waves look alike. When present, one precedes each QRS complex. |
| PR interval | 0.12-0.20 sec and constant from beat to beat |
| QRS duration | 0.10 sec or less unless an intraventricular conduction delay exists |

# Atrial Rhythms

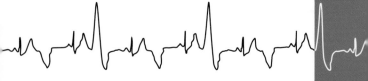

## INTRODUCTION

P waves reflect atrial depolarization. A rhythm that begins in the SA node has one positive (upright) P wave before each QRS complex. A rhythm that begins in the atria will have a positive P wave that is shaped differently than P waves that begin in the SA node. This difference in P wave configuration occurs because the impulse begins in the atria and follows a different conduction pathway to the AV node.

### Atrial Dysrhythmias: Mechanisms

Atrial dysrhythmias reflect abnormal electrical impulse formation and conduction in the atria. They result from altered automaticity, triggered activity, or reentry. Altered automaticity and triggered activity are disorders in impulse *formation*. Reentry is a disorder in impulse *conduction*. Dysrhythmias that result from disorders of impulse formation are often referred to as automatic. Dysrhythmias that result from a disorder in impulse conduction are referred to as reentrant.

## PREMATURE ATRIAL COMPLEXES (PACs)

A premature atrial complex (PAC) occurs when an irritable site (focus) within the atria fires before the next SA node impulse is due to fire (Figure 4-1). This interrupts the sinus rhythm. If the irritable site is close to the SA node, the atrial P wave will look very similar to the P waves initiated by the SA node. The P wave of a PAC may be biphasic (partly positive, partly negative), flattened, notched, or pointed. The ECG characteristics of PACs are shown in Table 4-1.

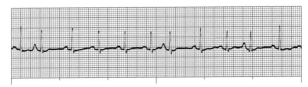

**Figure 4-1**    Sinus tachycardia with three PACs. (From the left, beats 2, 7, and 10 are PACs.)

| Table **4-1** | Characteristics of Premature Atrial Complexes (PACs) |
|---|---|
| Rate | Usually within normal range, but depends on underlying rhythm |
| Rhythm | Regular with premature beats |
| P waves | Premature (occurring earlier than the next expected sinus P wave), positive (upright) in lead II, one before each QRS complex, often differ in shape from sinus P waves—may be flattened, notched, pointed, biphasic, or lost in the preceding T wave |
| PR interval | May be normal or prolonged depending on the prematurity of the beat |
| QRS duration | Usually 0.10 sec or less but may be wide (aberrant) or absent, depending on the prematurity of the beat; the QRS of the PAC is similar in shape to those of the underlying rhythm unless the PAC is abnormally conducted |

## Noncompensatory vs. Compensatory Pause

A noncompensatory (incomplete) pause often follows a PAC. This represents the delay during which the SA node resets its rhythm for the next beat. A compensatory (complete) pause often follows premature ventricular complexes (PVCs). To find out whether or not the pause following a premature complex is compensatory or noncompensatory, measure the distance between three normal beats. Then compare that measurement to the distance between three beats, one of which includes the premature complex. The pause is *noncompensatory* if the normal beat following the premature complex occurs before it was expected (i.e., the period between the complex before and after the premature beat is less than two normal R-R intervals). The pause is *compensatory* if the normal beat following the premature complex occurs when expected (i.e., the period between the complex before and after the premature beat is the same as two normal R-R intervals).

## Aberrantly Conducted PACs

PACs associated with a wide QRS complex are called aberrantly conducted PACs. This indicates that conduction through the ventricles is abnormal (Figure 4-2).

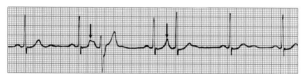

**Figure 4-2**    Premature atrial complexes with and without abnormal conduction (aberrancy).

## Nonconducted PACs

Sometimes, when a PAC occurs very early and close to the T wave of the preceding beat, only a P wave may be seen with no QRS after it (appearing as a pause) (Figure 4-3). This type of PAC is called a *nonconducted* or *blocked* PAC because the P wave occurred too early to be conducted.

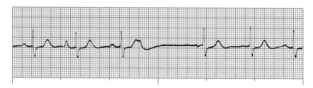

**Figure 4-3**    Sinus rhythm with a nonconducted (blocked) PAC.

# WANDERING ATRIAL PACEMAKER

Multiformed atrial rhythm is an updated term for the rhythm formerly known as wandering atrial pacemaker. With this rhythm, the size, shape, and direction of the P waves vary, sometimes from beat to beat. The difference in the look of the P waves is a result of the gradual shifting of the dominant pacemaker between the SA node, the atria, and/or the AV junction (Figure 4-4). The ECG characteristics of wandering atrial pacemaker are shown in Table 4-2.

Lead II (continuous)

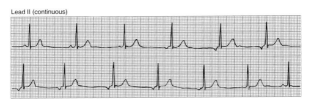

**Figure 4-4**  Wandering atrial pacemaker. Continuous strip (lead II).

| Table 4-2 | Characteristics of Wandering Atrial Pacemaker (Multiformed Atrial Rhythm) |
|---|---|
| Rate | Usually 60-100 beats/min, but may be slow; if the rate is greater than 100 beats/min, the rhythm is termed *multifocal* (or *chaotic*) *atrial tachycardia* |
| Rhythm | May be irregular as the pacemaker site shifts from the SA node to ectopic atrial locations and the AV junction |
| P waves | Size, shape, and direction may change from beat to beat; at least three different P wave configurations (seen in the same lead) are required for a diagnosis of wandering atrial pacemaker or multifocal atrial tachycardia |
| PR interval | Variable |
| QRS duration | 0.10 sec or less unless an intraventricular conduction delay exists |

## MULTIFOCAL ATRIAL TACHYCARDIA

When wandering atrial pacemaker is associated with a ventricular rate greater than 100 beats/min, the rhythm is called multifocal atrial tachycardia (MAT) (Figure 4-5). In MAT, multiple ectopic sites stimulate the atria.

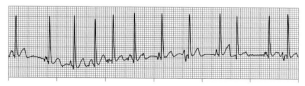

**Figure 4-5**  Multifocal atrial tachycardia (MAT), also known as chaotic atrial tachycardia. Premature atrial complexes (PACs) occur at varying cycle lengths and with differing shapes.

## SUPRAVENTRICULAR TACHYCARDIA (SVT)

Supraventricular arrhythmias (SVA) begin above the bifurcation of the bundle of His. This means that supraventricular arrhythmias include rhythms that begin in the SA node, atrial tissue, or the AV junction. The term supraventricular tachycardia (SVT) includes three main types of fast rhythms, which are illustrated in Figure 4-6.

- Atrial tachycardia (AT). In AT, an irritable site in the atria fires automatically at a rapid rate.
- AV nodal reentrant tachycardia (AVNRT). In AVNRT, fast and slow pathways in the AV node form an electrical circuit or loop. The impulse spins around the AV nodal (junctional) area.
- AV reentrant tachycardia (AVRT). In AVRT, the impulse begins above the ventricles but travels via a pathway other than the AV node and bundle of His.

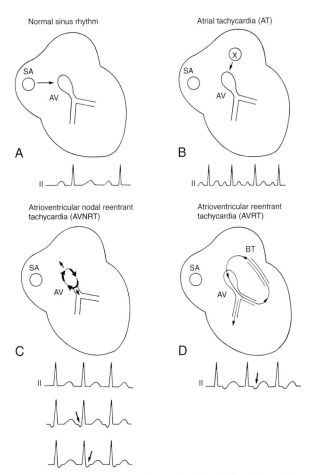

**Figure 4-6** Types of supraventricular tachycardias. **A,** Normal sinus rhythm is presented here as a reference. **B,** Atrial tachycardia. **C,** AV nodal reentrant tachycardia (AVNRT). **D,** AV reentrant tachycardia (AVRT). BT = bypass tract.

## ATRIAL TACHYCARDIA

Atrial tachycardia consists of a series of rapid beats from an irritable site in the atria. This rapid atrial rate overrides the SA node and becomes the pacemaker. Conduction of the atrial impulse to the ventricles is often 1:1. This means that every atrial impulse is conducted to the ventricles. Atrial tachycardia looks similar to sinus tachycardia but atrial P waves differ in shape from sinus P waves. An example of this rhythm is shown in Figure 4-7.

Atrial tachycardia that starts or ends suddenly is called paroxysmal atrial tachycardia (PAT). With very rapid atrial rates, the AV node begins to filter some of the impulses coming to it. By doing so it protects the ventricles from excessively rapid rates. When the AV node selectively filters conduction of some of these impulses, the rhythm is called paroxysmal atrial tachycardia with block.

- Atrial tachycardia that begins in a small area (focus) within the heart is called focal atrial tachycardia. There are several types of focal atrial tachycardia.
- Automatic atrial tachycardia (also called ectopic atrial tachycardia) is another type of AT. This type of AT often has a "warm up" period. This means there is a progressive shortening of the P-P interval for the first few beats of the arrhythmia. Automatic AT gradually slows down as it ends. This has been called a "cool down" period. The atrial rate is usually between 100 and 250 beats/min.

The ECG characteristics of atrial tachycardia are shown in Table 4-3.

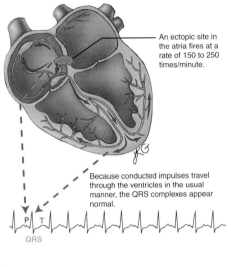

All the atrial impulses are conducted through the AV node. This results in a P wave preceding each QRS complex.

An ectopic site in the atria fires at a rate of 150 to 250 times/minute.

Because conducted impulses travel through the ventricles in the usual manner, the QRS complexes appear normal.

Although the P waves appear upright, they tend to look different from those seen when the impulse is initiated from the SA node.

P T
QRS

**Figure 4-7** Atrial tachycardia.

| Table **4-3** | Characteristics of Atrial Tachycardia |
|---|---|
| Rate | 100-250 beats/min |
| Rhythm | Regular |
| P waves | One positive P wave precedes each QRS complex in lead II; P waves differ in shape from sinus P waves; an isoelectric baseline is usually present between P waves |
| PR interval | May be shorter or longer than normal |
| QRS duration | 0.10 sec or less unless an intraventricular conduction delay exists |

## AV NODAL REENTRANT TACHYCARDIA (AVNRT)

AVNRT is caused by reentry in the area of the AV node. In the normal AV node, there is only one pathway through which an electrical impulse is conducted from the SA node to the ventricles. Patients with AVNRT have two conduction pathways within the AV node that conduct impulses at different speeds and recover at different rates. The fast pathway conducts impulses rapidly but has a long refractory period (slow recovery time). The slow pathway conducts impulses slowly but has a short refractory period (fast recovery time). Under the right conditions, the fast and slow pathways can form an electrical circuit or loop. As one side of the loop is recovering, the other is firing.

AVNRT is usually caused by a PAC that is spread by the electrical circuit. This allows the impulse to spin around in a circle indefinitely, reentering the normal electrical pathway with each pass around the circuit. The result is a very rapid and regular rhythm that ranges from 150 to 250 beats/min (Figure 4-8).

A regular, narrow-QRS tachycardia that starts or ends suddenly is called paroxysmal supraventricular tachycardia (PSVT) (Figure 4-9). P waves are seldom seen because they are hidden in T waves of preceding beats. The QRS is narrow unless there is a problem with conduction of the impulse through the ventricles, as in a bundle branch block. The ECG characteristics of AVNRT are summarized in Table 4-4.

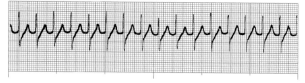

**Figure 4-8**     AV nodal reentrant tachycardia (AVNRT).

| Table 4-4 | Characteristics of AV Nodal Reentrant Tachycardia (AVNRT) |
|---|---|
| Rate | 150-250 beats/min |
| Rhythm | Ventricular rhythm is usually very regular |
| P waves | P waves are often hidden in the QRS complex. If the ventricles are stimulated first and then the atria, a negative (inverted) P wave will appear after the QRS in leads II, III, and aVF. When the atria are depolarized after the ventricles, the P wave typically distorts the end of the QRS complex. |
| PR interval | P waves are not seen before the QRS complex, therefore the PR interval is not measurable |
| QRS duration | 0.10 sec or less unless an intraventricular conduction delay exists |

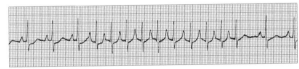

**Figure 4-9** Paroxysmal supraventricular tachycardia (PSVT).

## AV REENTRANT TACHYCARDIA (AVRT)

The next most common type of SVT is AV reentrant tachycardia (AVRT). AVRT involves a pathway of impulse conduction outside the AV node and bundle of His. Preexcitation is a term used to describe rhythms that originate from above the ventricles but in which the impulse travels via a pathway other than the AV node and bundle of His. As a result, the supraventricular impulse excites the ventricles earlier than would be expected if the impulse traveled by way of the normal conduction system. Patients with preexcitation syndromes are prone to AVRT.

In WPW syndrome, the PR interval is short (less than 0.12 sec) because the impulse travels very quickly across the accessory pathway, bypassing the normal delay in the AV node

(Figure 4-10). As the impulse crosses the insertion point of the accessory pathway in the ventricular muscle, that part of the ventricle is stimulated earlier (preexcited) than if the impulse had followed the normal conduction pathway through the bundle of His and Purkinje fibers. On the ECG, preexcitation of the ventricles can be seen as a delta wave in some leads. A delta wave is an initial slurring of the QRS complex. The direction of the ST-segment and T wave changes are usually opposite the direction of the delta wave and QRS complex. The ECG characteristics of WPW are summarized in Table 4-5.

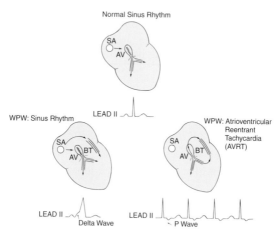

**Figure 4-10**  Conduction during sinus rhythm in the normal heart (*top*) spreads from the sinoatrial (SA) node to the atrioventricular (AV) node and then down the bundle branches. The jagged line indicates physiologic slowing of conduction in the AV node. With the WPW syndrome (*bottom left*), an abnormal accessory conduction pathway called a bypass tract (BT) connects the atria and ventricles. With WPW, during sinus rhythm, the electrical impulse is conducted quickly down the bypass tract, preexciting the ventricles before the impulse arrives via the AV node. Consequently, the P-R interval is short and the QRS complex is wide, with slurring at its onset (delta wave). WPW predisposes patients to develop an atrioventricular reentrant tachycardia (AVRT) (*bottom right*) in which a premature atrial beat may spread down the normal pathway to the ventricles, travel back up the bypass tract, and recirculate down the AV node again. This reentrant loop can repeat itself over and over, resulting in a tachycardia. Notice the normal QRS complex and often negative P wave in lead II during this type of bypass-tract tachycardia.

| Table 4-5 | Characteristics of Wolff-Parkinson-White (WPW) Syndrome |
|---|---|
| Rate | Usually 60-100 beats/min, if the underlying rhythm is sinus in origin |
| Rhythm | Regular, unless associated with atrial fibrillation |
| P waves | Normal and positive in lead II unless WPW is associated with atrial fibrillation |
| PR interval | If P waves are observed, less than 0.12 sec |
| QRS duration | Usually greater than 0.12 sec. Slurred upstroke of the QRS complex (delta wave) may be seen in one or more leads. |

## ATRIAL FLUTTER

Atrial flutter has been classified into two types:

- Type I atrial flutter is caused by reentry. In this type of atrial flutter, an impulse circles around a large area of tissue, such as the entire right atrium. Type I atrial flutter is also called typical or classical atrial flutter. In type I atrial flutter, the atrial rate ranges from 250 to 350 beats/min.
- Type II atrial flutter is called atypical or very rapid atrial flutter. The precise mechanism of type II atrial flutter has not been defined. Patients with this type of atrial flutter often develop atrial fibrillation. In type II atrial flutter, the atrial rate ranges from 350 to 450 beats/min.

If the AV node blocks the impulses coming to it at a regular rate, the resulting ventricular rhythm will be regular. If the AV node blocks the impulses at an irregular rate, the resulting ventricular rhythm will be irregular. An example of atrial flutter is shown in Figure 4-11. The ECG characteristics of atrial flutter are shown in Table 4-6.

## ATRIAL FIBRILLATION (AFib)

Atrial fibrillation (AFib) occurs because of irritable sites in the atria firing at a rate of 400 to 600 times per minute. These rapid impulses cause the muscles of the atria to quiver (fibrillate). This results in ineffectual atrial contraction, decreased stroke volume, a subsequent decrease in cardiac output, and loss of atrial kick. An example of atrial fibrillation is shown in Figure 4-12. The ECG characteristics of AFib are shown in Table 4-7.

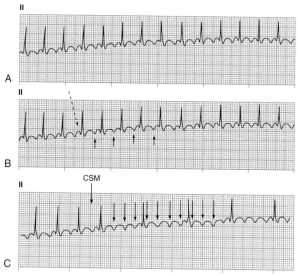

**Figure 4-11    A-C,** Atrial flutter. **A,** This rhythm strip shows a narrow-QRS tachycardia with a ventricular rate just under 150 beats/min. **B,** The same rhythm shown in **A** with arrows added indicating possible atrial activity. **C,** When carotid sinus massage (CSM) is performed, the rate of conduction through the AV node slows, revealing atrial flutter.

| Table 4-6 | Characteristics of Atrial Flutter |
|-----------|-----------------------------------|
| Rate | Atrial rate 250-450 beats/min, typically 300 beats/min; ventricular rate variable—determined by AV blockade; the ventricular rate will usually not exceed 180 beats/min due to the intrinsic conduction rate of the AV junction |
| Rhythm | Atrial regular, ventricular regular or irregular depending on AV conduction/blockade |
| P Waves | No identifiable P waves; saw-toothed "flutter" waves are present |
| PR interval | Not measurable |
| QRS Duration | 0.10 sec or less but may be widened if flutter waves are buried in the QRS complex or an intraventricular conduction delay exists |

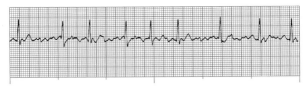

**Figure 4-12**   Atrial fibrillation with a ventricular response of 67 to 120 beats/min.

| Table 4-7 | Characteristics of Atrial Fibrillation |
|-----------|----------------------------------------|
| Rate | Atrial rate usually 400-600 beats/min; ventricular rate variable |
| Rhythm | Ventricular rhythm usually irregularly irregular |
| P waves | No identifiable P waves, fibrillatory waves present; erratic, wavy baseline |
| PR interval | Not measurable |
| QRS duration | 0.10 sec or less but may be widened if an intraventricular conduction delay exists |

# Junctional Rhythms

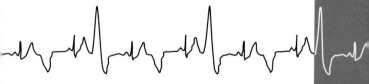

## INTRODUCTION

The AV node is a group of specialized cells located in the lower part of the right atrium, above the base of the tricuspid valve. The AV node's main job is to delay an electrical impulse. This allows the atria to contract and complete the filling of the ventricles with blood before the next ventricular contraction.

After passing through the AV node, the electrical impulse enters the bundle of His. The bundle of His is located in the upper part of the interventricular septum. It connects the AV node with the two bundle branches. The bundle of His has pacemaker cells that are capable of discharging at a rhythmic rate of 40 to 60 beats/min. The AV node and the nonbranching portion of the bundle of His are called the AV junction (Figure 5-1). The bundle of His conducts the electrical impulse to the right and left bundle branches.

Remember that the SA node is normally the heart's pacemaker. The AV junction may assume responsibility for pacing the heart if:

- The SA node fails to discharge (such as sinus arrest)
- An impulse from the SA node is generated but blocked as it exits the SA node (such as SA block)
- The rate of discharge of the SA node is slower than that of the AV junction (such as a sinus bradycardia or the slower phase of a sinus arrhythmia)

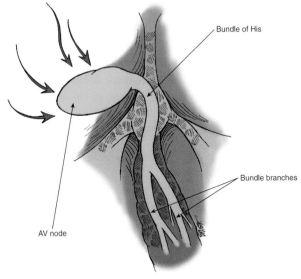

**Figure 5-1**    The AV junction.

- An impulse from the SA node is generated and is conducted through the atria but is not conducted to the ventricles (such as an AV block)

Rhythms that begin in the AV junction used to be called nodal rhythms until electrophysiologic studies proved the AV node does not contain pacemaker cells. The cells nearest the bundle of His are actually responsible for secondary pacing function. Rhythms originating from the AV junction are now called junctional dysrhythmias.

If the AV junction paces the heart, the electrical impulse must travel in a backward (retrograde) direction to activate the atria. If a P wave is seen, it will be inverted in leads II, III, and aVF because the impulse is traveling away from the positive electrode (Figure 5-2). If the atria depolarize before the ventricles, an inverted P wave will be seen *before* the QRS complex (Figure 5-3) and the PR interval will usually measure 0.12 second or less. The

PR interval is shorter than usual because an impulse that begins in the AV junction does not have to travel as far to stimulate the ventricles. If the atria and ventricles depolarize at the same time, a P wave will not be visible because it will be hidden in the QRS complex. If the atria depolarize after the ventricles, an inverted P wave will appear *after* the QRS complex.

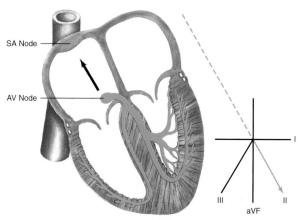

**Figure 5-2**    If the AV junction paces the heart, the electrical impulse must travel in a backward (retrograde) direction to activate the atria. If a P wave is seen, it will be inverted in leads II, III, and aVF because the impulse is traveling away from the positive electrode.

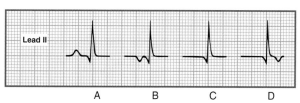

**Figure 5-3**    **A,** With a sinus rhythm, the P wave is positive (upright) in lead II because the wave of depolarization is moving toward the positive electrode. The P wave associated with a junctional beat (in lead II) may be: **B,** inverted (retrograde) and appear before the QRS; **C,** be hidden by the QRS; or **D,** appear after the QRS.

# PREMATURE JUNCTIONAL COMPLEXES (PJCS)

A premature junctional complex (PJC) occurs when an irritable site (focus) within the AV junction fires before the next SA node impulse is due to fire. This interrupts the sinus rhythm. Because the impulse is conducted through the ventricles in the usual manner, the QRS complex will usually measure 0.10 second or less. A noncompensatory (incomplete) pause often follows a PJC. This pause represents the delay during which the SA node resets its rhythm for the next beat.

Junctional complexes may come early (before the next expected sinus beat) or late (after the next expected sinus beat). If the complex is *early* it is called a premature junctional complex. If the complex is *late* it is called a junctional escape beat. To determine if a complex is early or late, you need to see at least two sinus beats in a row to establish the regularity of the underlying rhythm. Examples of PJCs are shown in Figure 5-4. The ECG characteristics of PJCs are shown in Table 5-1.

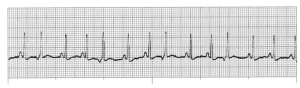

**Figure 5-4**  Sinus tachycardia at 136 beats/min with frequent PJCs.

| Table **5-1** | Characteristics of Premature Junctional Complexes (PJCs) |
| --- | --- |
| Rate | Usually within normal range, but depends on underlying rhythm |
| Rhythm | Regular with premature beats |
| P waves | May occur before, during, or after the QRS; if visible, the P wave is inverted in leads II, III, and aVF |
| PR interval | If a P wave occurs before the QRS, the PR interval will usually be 0.12 sec or less; if no P wave occurs before the QRS, there will be no PR interval |
| QRS duration | Usually 0.10 sec or less unless it is aberrantly conducted or an intraventricular conduction delay exists |

## JUNCTIONAL ESCAPE BEATS/RHYTHM

A junctional escape beat begins in the AV junction and appears *late* (after the next expected sinus beat). Junctional escape beats frequently occur during episodes of sinus arrest or follow pauses of nonconducted PACs. An example of a junctional escape beat is shown in Figure 5-5. The ECG characteristics of junctional escape beats are shown in Table 5-2.

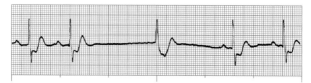

**Figure 5-5**    Sinus rhythm at 71 beats/min with a prolonged PR interval (0.24 sec), an episode of sinus arrest, a junctional escape beat, and ST-segment depression.

| Table **5-2** | Characteristics of Junctional Escape Beats |
|---|---|
| Rate | Usually within normal range, but depends on underlying rhythm |
| Rhythm | Regular with *late* beats |
| P waves | May occur before, during, or after the QRS; if visible, the P wave is inverted in leads II, III, and aVF |
| PR interval | If a P wave occurs before the QRS, the PR interval will usually be 0.12 sec or less; if no P wave occurs before the QRS, there will be no PR interval |
| QRS duration | Usually 0.10 sec or less unless it is aberrantly conducted or an intraventricular conduction delay exists |

A junctional *rhythm* is several sequential junctional escape *beats*. Remember that the intrinsic rate of the AV junction is 40 to 60 beats/min. Because a junctional rhythm starts from above the ventricles, the QRS complex is usually narrow and its rhythm is very regular. If the AV junction paces the heart at a rate slower than 40 beats/min, the resulting rhythm is called a junctional bradycardia. This may seem confusing because the AV junction's normal pacing rate (40-60 beats/min) *is* bradycardic. However, the term junctional bradycardia refers to a rate slower than normal for the AV junction. An example of a junctional rhythm is shown in Figure 5-6. The ECG characteristics of a junctional rhythm are shown in Table 5-3.

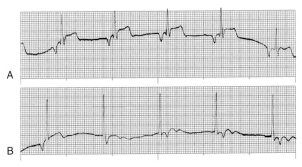

A

B

**Figure 5-6**  Junctional escape rhythm. Continuous strips. **A,** Note the inverted (retrograde) P waves before the QRS complexes. **B,** Note the change in the location of the P waves. In the first beat, the retrograde P wave is seen before the QRS. In the second beat, no P wave is seen. In the remaining beats, the P wave is seen after the QRS complexes.

| Table **5-3** | Characteristics of Junctional Escape Rhythm |
|---|---|
| Rate | 40-60 beats/min |
| Rhythm | Very regular |
| P waves | May occur before, during, or after the QRS; if visible, the P wave is inverted in leads II, III, and aVF |
| PR interval | If a P wave occurs before the QRS, the PR interval will usually be 0.12 sec or less; if no P wave occurs before the QRS, there will be no PR interval |
| QRS duration | Usually 0.10 sec or less unless it is aberrantly conducted or an intraventricular conduction delay exists |

## ACCELERATED JUNCTIONAL RHYTHM

If the AV junction speeds up and fires at a rate of 61 to 100 beats/min, the resulting rhythm is called an accelerated junctional rhythm. This rhythm is caused by enhanced automaticity of the bundle of His. The only ECG difference between a junctional rhythm and an accelerated junctional rhythm is the increase in the ventricular rate. An example of an accelerated junctional rhythm is shown in Figure 5-7. The ECG characteristics of this rhythm are shown in Table 5-4.

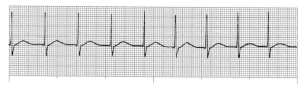

**Figure 5-7**    Accelerated junctional rhythm at 93 beats/min.

| Table 5-4 | Characteristics of Accelerated Junctional Rhythm |
|---|---|
| Rate | 61-100 beats/min |
| Rhythm | Very regular |
| P waves | May occur before, during, or after the QRS; if visible, the P wave is inverted in leads II, III, and aVF |
| PR interval | If a P wave occurs before the QRS, the PR interval will usually be 0.12 sec or less; if no P wave occurs before the QRS, there will be no PR interval |
| QRS duration | Usually 0.10 sec or less unless it is aberrantly conducted or an intraventricular conduction delay exists |

## JUNCTIONAL TACHYCARDIA

Junctional tachycardia is an ectopic rhythm that begins in the pacemaker cells found in the bundle of His. When three or more sequential PJCs occur at a rate of more than 100 beats/min, a junctional tachycardia exists. Nonparoxysmal (gradual onset) junctional tachycardia usually starts as an accelerated junctional rhythm but the heart rate gradually increases to more than 100 beats/min. The usual ventricular rate for nonparoxysmal junctional tachycardia is 101 to 140 beats/min. Paroxysmal junctional tachycardia starts and ends suddenly and is often precipitated by a PJC. The ventricular rate for paroxysmal junctional tachycardia is generally faster, 140 beats/min or more. An example of junctional tachycardia is shown in Figure 5-8. The ECG characteristics of this rhythm are shown in Table 5-5.

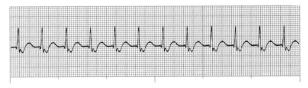

**Figure 5-8**   Junctional tachycardia at 120 beats/min.

| Table **5-5** | Characteristics of Junctional Tachycardia |
|---|---|
| Rate | 101-180 beats/min |
| Rhythm | Very regular |
| P waves | May occur before, during, or after the QRS; if visible, the P wave is inverted in leads II, III, and aVF |
| PR interval | If a P wave occurs before the QRS, the PR interval will usually be 0.12 sec or less; if no P wave occurs before the QRS, there will be no PR interval |
| QRS duration | Usually 0.10 sec or less unless it is aberrantly conducted or an intraventricular conduction delay exists |

# Ventricular Rhythms

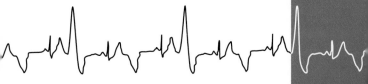

## INTRODUCTION

The ventricles are the heart's least efficient pacemaker. If the ventricles function as the heart's pacemaker, they normally generate impulses at a rate of 20 to 40 beats/min. The ventricles may assume responsibility for pacing the heart if:

- SA node fails to discharge
- Impulse from the SA node is generated but blocked as it exits the SA node
- Rate of discharge of the SA node is slower than that of the ventricles
- Irritable site in either ventricle produces an early beat or rapid rhythm

If an area of either ventricle becomes ischemic or injured, it can become irritable. This irritability affects the manner in which impulses are conducted. Ventricular beats and rhythms can start in any part of the ventricles and may occur as a result of reentry, enhanced automaticity, or triggered activity. When an ectopic site within a ventricle assumes responsibility for pacing the heart, the electrical impulse bypasses the normal intraventricular conduction pathway. This results in stimulation of the ventricles at slightly different times. As a result, ventricular beats and rhythms usually have QRS complexes that are abnormally shaped and longer than normal (greater than 0.12 sec).

## PREMATURE VENTRICULAR COMPLEXES (PVCs)

A premature ventricular complex (PVC) arises from an irritable site within either ventricle. PVCs may be caused by enhanced automaticity or reentry. By definition, a PVC is *premature*, occurring earlier than the next expected sinus beat. The QRS of a PVC is typically equal to or greater than 0.12 second because the PVC causes the ventricles to fire prematurely and in an abnormal manner (Figure 6-1). The T wave is usually in the opposite direction of the QRS complex. A full compensatory pause often follows a PVC.

   A fusion beat (Figure 6-2) is a result of an electrical impulse from a supraventricular site (such as the SA node) discharging at the same time as an ectopic site in the ventricles. Because fusion beats are a result of both supraventricular and ventricular depolarization, these beats do not resemble normally conducted beats, nor do they resemble true ventricular beats.

### Types of PVCs
### Uniform and Multiformed PVCs
Premature ventricular beats that look the same in the same lead and begin from the same anatomic site (focus) are called uniform PVCs (Figure 6-3). PVCs that look different from one another in the same lead are called multiform PVCs (Figure 6-4).

### Interpolated PVCs
A PVC may occur without interfering with the normal cardiac cycle. An interpolated PVC (Figure 6-5) does not have a full compensatory pause. It is "squeezed" between two regular complexes and does not disturb the underlying rhythm. The PR interval of the cardiac cycle following the PVC may be longer than normal.

### R-on-T PVCs
R-on-T PVCs occur when the R wave of a PVC falls on the T wave of the preceding beat (Figure 6-6).

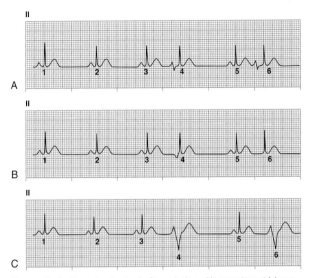

A

B

C

**Figure 6-1** Premature beats. **A,** Sinus rhythm with premature atrial complexes. The fourth and sixth beats are preceded by premature P waves that look different from the normally conducted sinus beats. Note that the QRS complex that follows each of these PACs is narrow and identical in appearance to that of the sinus-conducted beats. **B,** Sinus rhythm with premature junctional complexes. The fourth and sixth beats are PJCs. Beat No. 4 is preceded by an inverted P wave with a short PR interval. There is no identifiable atrial activity associated with beat No. 6. **C,** Sinus rhythm with premature ventricular complexes. The fourth and sixth beats are very different in appearance from the normally conducted sinus beats. Beats 4 and 6 are PVCs. They are not preceded by P waves.

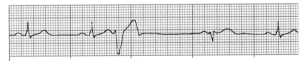

**Figure 6-2** Sinus bradycardia with a PVC (third complex from the left) and a fusion beat (fourth complex from the left).

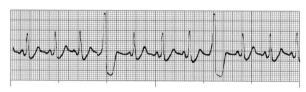

**Figure 6-3**    Sinus tachycardia with frequent uniform PVCs.

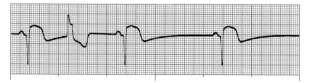

**Figure 6-4**    Sinus tachycardia with multiform PVCs.

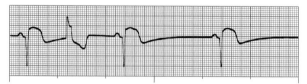

**Figure 6-5**    Sinus bradycardia with an interpolated PVC and ST-segment elevation.

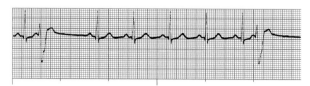

**Figure 6-6**    Sinus rhythm with two R-on-T PVCs.

## Paired PVCs (Couplets)

Two PVCs in a row are called a couplet or paired PVCs (Figure 6-7). The appearance of couplets indicates the ventricular ectopic site is very irritable. Three or more PVCs in a row at a rate of more than 100 beats/min is considered a "salvo," "run," or "burst" of ventricular tachycardia. The general characteristics of PVCs are shown in Table 6-1.

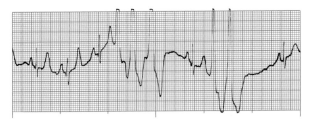

**Figure 6-7**  Sinus rhythm with a run of VT and one episode of couplets.

| Table **6-1** | Characteristics of Premature Ventricular Complexes (PVCs) |
|---|---|
| Rate | Usually within normal range, but depends on underlying rhythm |
| Rhythm | Essentially regular with premature beats; if the PVC is an interpolated PVC, the rhythm will be regular |
| P waves | Usually absent or, with retrograde conduction to the atria, may appear after the QRS (usually upright in the ST-segment or T wave) |
| PR interval | None with the PVC because the ectopic originates in the ventricles |
| QRS duration | Greater than 0.12 sec, wide and bizarre; T wave usually in opposite direction of the QRS complex |

## VENTRICULAR ESCAPE BEATS/RHYTHM

Remember that premature beats are *early* and escape beats are *late*. In order to determine if a complex is early or late, we need to see at least two sinus beats in a row to establish the regularity of the underlying rhythm. Although ventricular escape beats share some of the same physical characteristics as PVCs (wide QRS complexes, T waves deflected in a direction opposite the QRS), they differ in some very important areas.

- A PVC appears *early*, before the next expected sinus beat. PVCs often reflect irritability in some area of the ventricles. When PVCs cause serious symptoms, medications are sometimes used to reduce the frequency with which they occur or eliminate them completely.

- A ventricular escape beat occurs after a pause in which a supraventricular pacemaker failed to fire. Thus the escape beat is *late*, appearing after the next expected sinus beat. A ventricular escape beat is a *protective* mechanism. It protects the heart from more extreme slowing or even asystole. Because it is protective, you would not want to administer any medication that would "wipe out" the escape beat.

An example of a ventricular escape beat is shown in Figure 6-8. The ECG characteristics of ventricular escape beats are shown in Table 6-2.

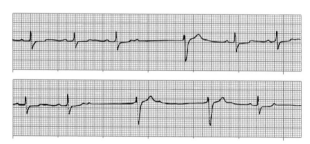

**Figure 6-8** Sinus rhythm with a prolonged PR interval, ST-segment depression. Note the ventricular escape beats following nonconducted premature atrial complexes.

| Table **6-2** | Characteristics of Ventricular Escape Beats |
|---|---|
| Rate | Usually within normal range, but depends on underlying rhythm |
| Rhythm | Essentially regular with late beats; the ventricular escape beat occurs *after* the next expected sinus beat |
| P waves | Usually absent or, with retrograde conduction to the atria, may appear after the QRS (usually upright in the ST-segment or T wave) |
| PR interval | None with the ventricular escape beat because the ectopic beat originates in the ventricles |
| QRS duration | Greater than 0.12 sec, wide and bizarre, T wave frequently in opposite direction of the QRS complex |

A ventricular escape or idioventricular rhythm (IVR) exists when three or more ventricular escape beats occur in a row at a rate of 20 to 40 beats/min. This rate is the intrinsic firing rate of the ventricles. The QRS complexes seen in IVR are wide and bizarre because the impulses begin in the ventricles, bypassing the normal conduction pathway. When the ventricular rate slows to a rate of less than 20 beats/min, some refer to the rhythm as an *agonal rhythm* or "dying heart." An example of IVR is shown in Figure 6-9. The characteristics of this rhythm are described in Table 6-3.

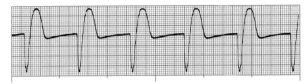

**Figure 6-9**    Idioventricular rhythm (IVR) at 35 beats/min.

| Table 6-3 | Characteristics of Idioventricular Rhythm (IVR) |
|---|---|
| Rate | 20-40 beats/min |
| Rhythm | Essentially regular |
| P waves | Usually absent or, with retrograde conduction to the atria, may appear after the QRS (usually upright in the ST-segment or T wave) |
| PR interval | None |
| QRS duration | Greater than 0.12 sec, T wave frequently in opposite direction of the QRS complex |

*ECG Pearl*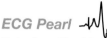

**Pulseless Electrical Activity**

Pulseless electrical activity (PEA) is a clinical situation, not a specific dysrhythmia. PEA exists when organized electrical activity (other than VT) is observed on the cardiac monitor, but the patient is unresponsive, apneic, and a pulse cannot be felt. Many conditions may cause PEA. PATCH-4-MD can be used as an aid in memorizing some of the possible causes of PEA.

- **P**ulmonary embolism
- **A**cidosis
- **T**ension pneumothorax
- **C**ardiac tamponade
- **H**ypovolemia (common cause of PEA)
- **H**ypoxia
- **H**eat/cold (hypothermia/hyperthermia)
- **H**ypokalemia/hyperkalemia (and other electrolytes)
- **M**yocardial infarction
- **D**rug overdose/accident

PEA has a poor prognosis unless the underlying cause can be rapidly identified and appropriately managed. Treatment includes CPR, oxygen, possible placement of an advanced airway, starting an IV, an aggressive search for possible causes of the situation, and medications per current resuscitation guidelines.

## ACCELERATED IDIOVENTRICULAR RHYTHM (AIVR)

An accelerated idioventricular rhythm (AIVR) exists when three or more ventricular escape beats occur in a row at a rate of 41 to 100 beats/min (Figure 6-10). AIVR is usually considered a benign escape rhythm that appears when the sinus rate slows and disappears when the sinus rate speeds up. Episodes of AIVR usually last a few seconds to a minute. Fusion beats are often seen at the onset and end of the rhythm. The ECG characteristics of AIVR are shown in Table 6-4.

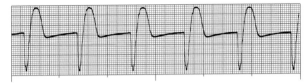

**Figure 6-10**   Accelerated idioventricular rhythm (AIVR) at 56 beats/min.

| Table **6-4** | Characteristics of Accelerated Idioventricular Rhythm (AIVR) |
|---|---|
| Rate | 41-100 beats/min |
| Rhythm | Essentially regular |
| P waves | Usually absent or, with retrograde conduction to the atria, may appear after the QRS (usually upright in the ST-segment or T wave) |
| PR interval | None |
| QRS duration | Greater than 0.12 sec, T wave frequently in opposite direction of the QRS complex |

## VENTRICULAR TACHYCARDIA (VT)

Ventricular tachycardia (VT) exists when three or more PVCs occur in a row at a rate greater than 100 beats/min. If VT occurs as a short run lasting less than 30 seconds, it is called *nonsustained VT* (Figure 6-11). When VT persists for more than 30 seconds it is called *sustained VT* (Figure 6-12).

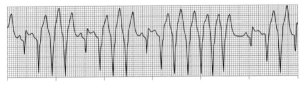

**Figure 6-11**   Nonsustained ventricular tachycardia. (Crawford MV, Spence MI: *Common sense approach to coronary care,* revised ed 6, St Louis, 1994, Mosby.)

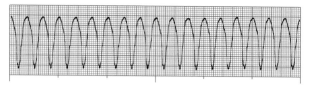

**Figure 6-12**   If this rhythm lasts longer than 30 seconds, it is called sustained ventricular tachycardia.

## Monomorphic VT

VT, like PVCs, may originate from an ectopic focus in either ventricle. When the QRS complexes of VT are of the same shape and amplitude, the rhythm is called **monomorphic VT** (Figure 6-13). Monomorphic VT with a ventricular rate greater than 200 beats/min is called ventricular flutter by some cardiologists. The ECG characteristics of monomorphic VT are shown in Table 6-5.

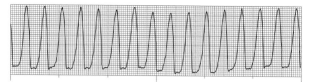

**Figure 6-13**   Monomorphic ventricular tachycardia.

| Table **6-5** | Characteristics of Monomorphic Ventricular Tachycardia |
|---|---|
| Rate | 101-250 beats/min |
| Rhythm | Essentially regular |
| P waves | May be present or absent; if present, they have no set relationship to the QRS complexes appearing between the QRSs at a rate different from that of the VT |
| PR interval | None |
| QRS duration | Greater than 0.12 sec; often difficult to differentiate between the QRS and T wave |

## Polymorphic VT

When the QRS complexes of VT vary in shape and amplitude from beat to beat, the rhythm is called **polymorphic VT** (Figure 6-14). In polymorphic VT, the QRS complexes appear to twist from upright to negative or negative to upright and back.

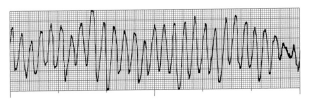

**Figure 6-14**   Polymorphic ventricular tachycardia. This rhythm strip is from a 77-year-old man 3 days post myocardial infarction (MI). His chief complaint at the onset of this episode was chest pain. He had a past medical history of a previous MI and an abdominal aortic aneurysm repair. The patient was given lidocaine and defibrillated several times without success. Lab work revealed a serum potassium (K+) level of 2.0. IV K+ was administered and the patient converted to a sinus rhythm with the next defibrillation.

Polymorphic VT is divided into two classifications based on its association with a normal or prolonged QT interval:

1. Normal QT
2. Long QT syndrome (LQTS)
   a. Acquired (iatrogenic)
   b. Congenital (idiopathic)

Polymorphic VT that occurs in the presence of a long QT interval is called Torsades de Pointes (TdP). *Torsades de pointes* is French for "twisting of the points," which describes the QRS that changes in shape, amplitude, and width and appears to "twist" around the isoelectric line, resembling a spindle. Polymorphic VT that occurs in the presence of a normal QT interval is simply referred to as *polymorphic VT* or *polymorphic VT resembling torsades de pointes.*

Long QT syndrome (LQTS) is an abnormality of the heart's electrical system. The mechanical function of the heart is entirely normal. The electrical problem is caused by defects in sodium and potassium channels that affect repolarization. These electrical defects prolong the QT interval, predisposing affected persons to TdP. The ECG characteristics of polymorphic VT are shown in Table 6-6.

| Table **6-6** | Characteristics of Polymorphic Ventricular Tachycardia |
|---|---|
| Rate | 150-300 beats/min, typically 200-250 beats/min |
| Rhythm | May be regular or irregular |
| P waves | None |
| PR interval | None |
| QRS duration | Greater than 0.12 sec; gradual alteration in amplitude and direction of the QRS complexes; a typical cycle consists of 5-20 QRS complexes |

## VENTRICULAR FIBRILLATION (VF)

Ventricular fibrillation (VF) is a chaotic rhythm that begins in the ventricles. In VF, there is no organized depolarization of the ventricles. The ventricular muscle quivers. As a result, there is no effective myocardial contraction and no pulse. The resulting rhythm looks chaotic with deflections that vary in shape and amplitude. No normal-looking waveforms are visible. VF with waves that are 3 or more mm high is called "coarse" VF (Figure 6-15). VF with low amplitude waves (less than 3 mm) is called "fine" VF (Figure 6-16). The ECG characteristics of VF are shown in Table 6-7. A comparison of ventricular arrhythmias is shown in Figure 6-17.

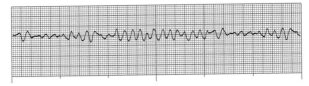

**Figure 6-15**   Coarse ventricular fibrillation.

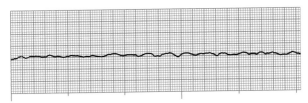

**Figure 6-16**   Fine ventricular fibrillation.

| Table **6-7** | Characteristics of Ventricular Fibrillation (VF) |
|---|---|
| Rate | Cannot be determined because there are no discernible waves or complexes to measure |
| Rhythm | Rapid and chaotic with no pattern or regularity |
| P waves | Not discernible |
| PR interval | Not discernible |
| QRS duration | Not discernible |

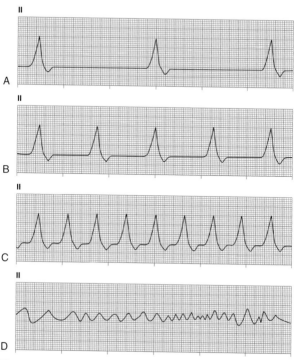

**Figure 6-17**    Comparison of ventricular arrhythmias. **A,** Idioventricular rhythm at 38 beats/min. **B,** Accelerated idioventricular rhythm at 75 beats/min. **C,** Monomorphic ventricular tachycardia at 150 beats/min. **D,** Coarse ventricular fibrillation.

*ECG Pearl*

**Cardiac Arrest Rhythms**
- Ventricular fibrillation
- (Pulseless) ventricular tachycardia
- Asystole
- Pulseless electrical activity

# ASYSTOLE (CARDIAC STANDSTILL)

Asystole is a total absence of ventricular electrical activity (Figure 6-18). There is no ventricular rate or rhythm, no pulse, and no cardiac output. Some atrial electrical activity may be evident. If atrial electrical activity is present, the rhythm is called "P wave" asystole (Figure 6-19). The ECG characteristics of asystole are shown in Table 6-8.

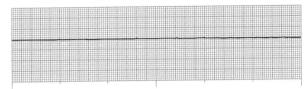

**Figure 6-18**    Asystole.

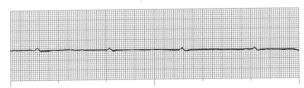

**Figure 6-19**    "P wave" asystole.

| Table 6-8 | Characteristics of Asystole |
|---|---|
| Rate | Ventricular usually not discernible but atrial activity may be seen ("P wave" asystole) |
| Rhythm | Ventricular not discernible, atrial may be discernible |
| P waves | Usually not discernible |
| PR interval | Not measurable |
| QRS duration | Absent |

# Atrioventricular (AV) Blocks

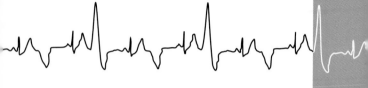

## INTRODUCTION

The AV junction is an area of specialized conduction tissue that provides the electrical links between the atrium and ventricle. If a delay or interruption in impulse conduction occurs within the AV node, bundle of His, or His-Purkinje system, the resulting dysrhythmia is called an atrioventricular (AV) block. AV blocks have been traditionally classified in two ways according to the degree of block and/or according to the site of the block.

Remember that the PR interval reflects depolarization of the right and left atria (P wave) and the spread of the impulse through the AV node, bundle of His, right and left bundle branches, and the Purkinje fibers. The PR interval is the key to differentiating the *type* of AV block. The key to differentiating the *level* (location) of the block is the width of the QRS complex and, in second- and third-degree AV blocks, the rate of the escape rhythm.

In first-degree AV block, impulses from the SA node to the ventricles are *delayed* (not blocked). First-degree AV block usually occurs at the AV node (Figure 7-1). With second-degree AV blocks, there is an *intermittent* disturbance in conduction of impulses between the atria and ventricles. The site of block in second-degree AV block type I is typically at the AV node. The site of block in second-degree AV block type II is the bundle of

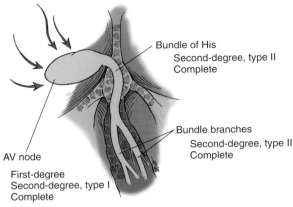

**Figure 7-1** Locations of AV block.

His or, more commonly, the bundle branches. In third-degree AV block, there is a *complete* block in conduction of impulses between the atria and ventricles. The site of block in a third-degree AV block may be the AV node or, more commonly, the bundle of His or bundle branches (Table 7-1).

*ECG Pearl*

The clinical significance of an AV block depends on:
- The degree (severity) of the block
- The rate of the escape pacemaker (junctional vs. ventricular)
- The patient's response to that ventricular rate

## FIRST-DEGREE AV BLOCK

A PR interval of normal duration (0.12 to 0.20 sec) indicates the electrical impulse was conducted normally through the atria, AV node, bundle of His, bundle branches, and Purkinje fibers. In first-degree AV block, all components of the ECG tracing are usually within normal limits except the PR interval. This is

| Table **7-1** | Classification of AV Blocks |
|---|---|

**CLASSIFICATION BY DEGREE**

| Name of Block | Type of Block |
|---|---|
| First-degree AV block | Incomplete |
| Second-degree AV block type I | Incomplete |
| Second-degree AV block type II | Incomplete |
| Third-degree AV block | Complete |

**CLASSIFICATION BY SITE/LOCATION**

| Site | Name of Block |
|---|---|
| AV node | First-degree AV block |
| | Second-degree AV block type I |
| | Third-degree AV block |
| **Infranodal (subnodal)** | |
| Bundle of His | Second-degree AV block type II (uncommon) |
| | Third-degree AV block |
| Bundle branches | Second-degree AV block type II (more common) |
| | Third-degree AV block |

because electrical impulses travel normally from the SA node through the atria, but there is a delay in impulse conduction, usually at the level of the AV node. Despite its name, in first-degree AV block, the sinus impulse is not blocked (all sinus beats are conducted)—impulses are *delayed* for the same period before they are conducted to the ventricles. This delay in AV conduction results in a PR interval that is longer than normal (more than 0.20 sec in duration) and constant (Figure 7-2). The ECG characteristics of first-degree AV block are shown in Table 7-2.

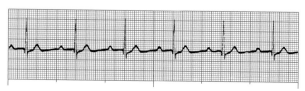

**Figure 7-2**    Sinus rhythm at 60 beats/min with a first-degree AV block.

| Table **7-2** | Characteristics of First-Degree AV Block |
|---|---|
| Rate | Usually within normal range, but depends on underlying rhythm |
| Rhythm | Regular |
| P waves | Normal in size and shape, one positive (upright) P wave before each QRS in leads II, III, and aVF |
| PR interval | Prolonged (greater than 0.20 sec) but constant |
| QRS duration | Usually 0.10 sec or less unless an intraventricular conduction delay exists |

## SECOND-DEGREE AV BLOCKS

### Overview

When some, but not all, atrial impulses are blocked from reaching the ventricles, second-degree AV block results. Because the SA node is generating impulses in a normal manner, each P wave will occur at a regular interval across the rhythm strip (all P waves will plot through on time), although not every P wave will be followed by a QRS complex. This suggests that the atria are being depolarized normally, but not every impulse is being conducted to the ventricles. As a result, more P waves than QRS complexes are seen on the ECG. Second-degree AV block is classified as type I or type II, depending on the location of the block. Second-degree AV block type I occurs above the bundle of His. Second-degree AV block type II occurs within or below the bundle of His.

### Second-Degree AV Block Type I (Wenckebach, Mobitz Type I)

The conduction delay in second-degree AV block type I usually occurs at the level of the AV node. An example of this type of AV block in Figure 7-3. ECG characteristics of second-degree AV Block type I are shown in Table 7-3.

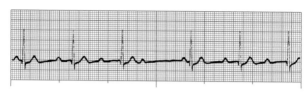

**Figure 7-3**    Second-degree AV block type I at 43 to 60 beats/min.

| Table **7-3** | Characteristics of Second-Degree AV Block Type I |
|---|---|
| Rate | Atrial rate is greater than the ventricular rate |
| Rhythm | Atrial regular (Ps plot through on time); ventricular irregular |
| P waves | Normal in size and shape; some P waves are not followed by a QRS complex (more Ps than QRSs) |
| PR interval | Lengthens with each cycle (although lengthening may be very slight), until a P wave appears without a QRS complex; the PRI *after* the nonconducted beat is shorter than the interval preceding the nonconducted beat |
| QRS duration | Usually 0.10 sec or less but is periodically dropped |

## Second-Degree AV Block, Type II (Mobitz Type II)

The conduction delay in second-degree AV block type II occurs below the AV node, either at the bundle of His or, more commonly, at the level of the bundle branches. This type of block is more serious than second-degree AV block type I and frequently progresses to third-degree AV block. An example of second-degree AV block type II is shown in Figure 7-4. The ECG characteristics of second-degree AV block type II are shown in Table 7-4.

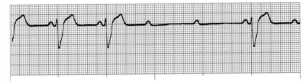

**Figure 7-4**    Second-degree AV block type II at 20 to 60 beats/min, ST segment elevation.

| Table 7-4 | Characteristics of Second-Degree AV Block Type II |
|---|---|
| Rate | Atrial rate is greater than the ventricular rate; ventricular rate is often slow |
| Rhythm | Atrial regular (Ps plot through on time), ventricular irregular |
| P waves | Normal in size and shape; some P waves are not followed by a QRS complex (more Ps than QRSs) |
| PR interval | Within normal limits or slightly prolonged but constant for the conducted beats; there may be some shortening of the PR interval that follows a nonconducted P wave |
| QRS duration | Usually 0.10 sec or greater, periodically absent after P waves |

## Second-Degree AV Block, 2:1 Conduction (2:1 AV Block)

You have learned that there are differences in the PR interval patterns in second-degree AV block type I and type II. In order to see compare PR intervals, we must see two PQRST cycles in a row. If there are more P waves than QRSs and the P waves occur on time, you now know that you have some type of AV block. If you then look at the PR intervals, you can begin to differentiate what type of AV block it is. For example, if the PR intervals get progressively longer and then a P wave appears with no QRS after it, you know that the rhythm is a second-degree AV block type I. If the PR intervals remain the same (constant) before the conducted beats, you know that the rhythm is a second-degree AV block type II. The QRS complex in a second-degree AV block type I is usually narrow. It is usually wide in a second-degree AV block type II.

In 2:1 AV block, two P waves occur for every one QRS complex (2:1 conduction). Since there are no two PQRST cycles in a row from which to compare PR intervals, the decision as to what to term the rhythm is based on the width of the QRS complex. A 2:1 AV block associated with a narrow QRS complex (0.10 sec or less) usually represents a form of second-degree AV block, type I (Figure 7-5). A 2:1 AV block associated with wide QRS complexes (greater than 0.10 sec) is usually associated with a delay in conduction below the bundle of His—thus it is usually a type II block (Figure 7-6).

A comparison of the types of second-degree AV blocks is shown in Figure 7-7. The ECG characteristics of 2:1 AV block are summarized in Table 7-5.

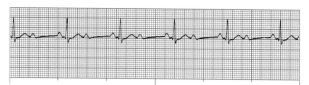

**Figure 7-5**   Second-degree AV block, 2:1 conduction, probably type I.

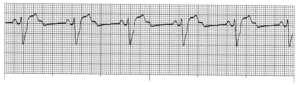

**Figure 7-6**   Second-degree AV block, 2:1 conduction, probably type II.

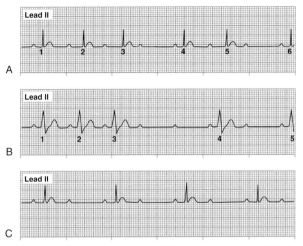

A

B

C

**Figure 7-7**    Types of second-degree AV block. **A,** Second-degree AV block type I. **B,** Second-degree AV block type II. **C,** Second-degree AV block 2:1 conduction.

| Table 7-5 | Characteristics of Second-Degree AV Block 2:1 Conduction (2:1 AV Block) |
|---|---|
| Rate | Atrial rate is twice the ventricular rate |
| Rhythm | Atrial regular (Ps plot through on time), ventricular regular |
| P waves | Normal in size and shape; every other P wave is followed by a QRS complex (more Ps than QRSs) |
| PR interval | Constant |
| QRS duration | Within normal limits, if the block occurs above the bundle of His (probably type I); wide if the block occurs below the bundle of His (probably type II); absent after every other P wave |

*ECG Pearl*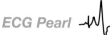

**A Quick Look at P Waves and AV Blocks**

| AV Block | P wave conduction |
|---|---|
| First-degree | All P waves conducted but delayed |
| Second-degree | Some P waves conducted, others blocked |
| Third-degree | No P waves conducted |

## THIRD-DEGREE AV BLOCK

Second-degree AV blocks are types of *incomplete* blocks because the AV junction conducts at least some impulses to the ventricles. In third-degree AV block, impulses generated by the SA node are blocked before reaching the ventricles so no P waves are conducted. The atria and ventricles beat independently of each other. Thus third-degree AV block is also called *complete* AV block. The block may occur at the AV node, bundle of His, or bundle branches. A secondary pacemaker (either junctional or ventricular) stimulates the ventricles; therefore, the QRS may be narrow or wide, depending on the location of the escape pacemaker and the condition of the intraventricular conduction system.

Third-degree AV block associated with an inferior MI is thought to be the result of a block above the bundle of His. It often occurs after progression from first-degree AV block or second-degree AV block type I. The resulting rhythm is usually stable because the escape pacemaker is usually junctional (narrow QRS complexes) with a ventricular rate of more than 40 beats/min (Figure 7-8).

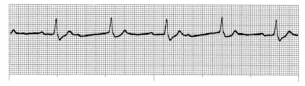

**Figure 7-8**    Third-degree AV block with a junctional escape pacemaker (QRS 0.08 to 0.10 sec).

Third-degree AV block associated with an anterior MI is usually preceded by second-degree AV block type II or an intraventricular conduction delay (right or left bundle branch block). The resulting rhythm is usually unstable because the escape pacemaker is usually ventricular (wide QRS complexes) with a ventricular rate of less than 40 beats/min (Figure 7-9). The ECG characteristics of third-degree AV block are shown in Table 7-6.

Table 7-7 will help you learn to recognize the differences between second- and third-degree AV blocks.

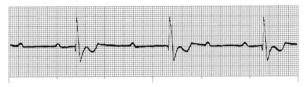

**Figure 7-9**  Third-degree AV block with a ventricular escape pacemaker (QRS 0.12 to 0.14 sec).

| Table 7-6 | Characteristics of Third-Degree AV Block |
| --- | --- |
| Rate | Atrial rate is greater than the ventricular rate; ventricular rate determined by origin of the escape rhythm |
| Rhythm | Atrial regular (Ps plot through on time), ventricular regular; there is no relationship between the atrial and ventricular rhythms |
| P waves | Normal in size and shape |
| PR interval | None—the atria and ventricles beat independently of each other, thus there is no true PR interval |
| QRS duration | Narrow or wide depending on the location of the escape pacemaker and the condition of the intraventricular conduction system; narrow = junctional pacemaker, wide = ventricular pacemaker |

| Table **7-7** | AV Blocks – Quick Summary | |
|---|---|---|
| | Second-Degree AV Block Type I | Second-Degree AV Block Type II |
| Ventricular rhythm | Irregular | Irregular |
| PR interval | Progressively lengthening | Constant |
| QRS width | Usually narrow | Usually wide |
| | **Second-Degree AV Block 2:1 Conduction** | **Third-Degree (Complete) AV Block** |
| Ventricular rhythm | Regular | Regular |
| PR interval | Constant | None—no relationship between P waves and QRS complexes |
| QRS width | May be narrow or wide | May be narrow or wide |

# Pacemaker Rhythms

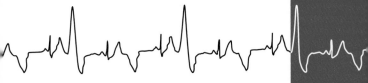

## PACEMAKER SYSTEMS

### Introduction

A pacemaker is an artificial pulse generator that delivers an electrical current to the heart to stimulate depolarization. Pacemaker systems are usually named according to where the electrodes are located and the route the electrical current takes to the heart. A pacemaker system (Figure 8-1) consists of a pulse generator (power source) and pacing lead(s). The pulse generator houses a battery and electronic circuitry. The circuitry works like a computer, converting energy from the battery into electrical pulses. A pacing lead is an insulated wire used to carry an electrical impulse from the pacemaker to the patient's heart. It also carries information about the heart's electrical activity back to the pacemaker. The exposed portion of the pacing lead is called an *electrode*, which is placed in direct contact with the heart.

### Permanent Pacemakers

A permanent pacemaker is implanted in the body, usually under local anesthesia. Pacemaker wires are surrounded by plastic catheters. The pacemaker's circuitry is housed in a hermetically sealed case made of titanium that is air-tight and impermeable to fluid.

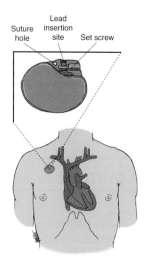

**Figure 8-1**   Permanent pacemaker.

## Temporary Pacemakers

Temporary pacing can be accomplished through transvenous, epicardial, or transcutaneous means.

- Transvenous pacemakers stimulate the endocardium of the right atrium or ventricle (or both) by means of an electrode introduced into a central vein, such as the subclavian or cephalic vein.
- Epicardial pacing is the placement of pacing leads directly onto or through the epicardium under direct visualization. Epicardial leads may be used when a patient is undergoing surgery and the outer surface of the heart is easy to reach. They are frequently used in neonates, children, and adolescents because of cardiac anatomy, small body size, and/or difficulty accessing the superior vena cava.
- Transcutaneous pacing (TCP) delivers pacing impulses to the heart using electrodes placed on the patient's thorax. TCP is also called *temporary external pacing* or *noninvasive pacing*.

## Pacemaker Electrodes

### Unipolar Electrodes

There are two types of pacemaker electrodes—unipolar and bipolar. A unipolar electrode (Figure 8-2) has one pacing electrode that is located at its distal tip. The negative electrode is in contact with the heart, and the pulse generator (located outside the heart) functions as the positive electrode. The pacemaker spikes produced by a unipolar electrode are often large because of the distance between the positive and negative electrodes.

### Bipolar Electrodes

A bipolar pacemaker electrode contains a positive and negative electrode at the distal tip of the pacing lead wire. Most temporary transvenous pacemakers have bipolar electrodes. A permanent pacemaker may have either a bipolar or a unipolar electrode. The spike produced by a bipolar electrode is often small and difficult to see.

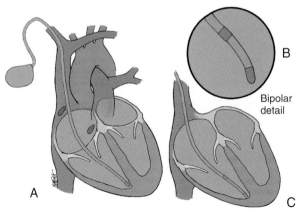

**Figure 8-2**    **A,** Unipolar pacemaker electrodes; **B** and **C,** bipolar pacemaker electrodes.

## Pacemaker Modes

### Fixed-Rate (Asynchronous) Pacemakers

A fixed-rate pacemaker continuously discharges at a preset rate (usually 70-80/min) regardless of the patient's heart rate. An advantage of the fixed-rate pacemaker is its simple circuitry, reducing the risk of pacemaker failure. However, this type of pacemaker does not sense the patient's own cardiac rhythm. This may result in competition between the patient's cardiac rhythm and that of the pacemaker. VT or VF may be induced if the pacemaker were to fire during the T wave (vulnerable period) of a preceding patient beat. Fixed-rate pacemakers are not often used today.

### Demand (Synchronous, Noncompetitive) Pacemakers

A demand pacemaker discharges only when the patient's heart rate drops below the pacemaker's preset (base) rate. For example, if the demand pacemaker was preset at a rate of 70 impulses/min, it would sense the patient's heart rate and allow electrical impulses to flow from the pacemaker through the pacing lead to stimulate the heart only when the rate fell below 70 beats/min. Demand pacemakers can be program-mable or nonprogrammable. The voltage level and impulse rate are preset at the time of manufacture in nonprogram-mable pacemakers.

## Pacemaker Identification Codes

Pacemaker identification codes are used to assist in identifying a pacemaker's preprogrammed pacing, sensing, and response functions (Table 8-1).

## Single-Chamber Pacemakers

A pacemaker that paces a single heart chamber (either the atrium or ventricle) has one lead placed in the heart. Atrial pacing is achieved by placing the pacing electrode in the right atrium. Stimulation of the atria produces a pacemaker spike on the ECG, followed by a P wave

| Table 8-1 | Pacemaker Codes | | | |
|---|---|---|---|---|
| Chamber Paced (First Letter) | Chamber Sensed (Second Letter) | Response to Sensing (Third Letter) | Programmable Functions (Fourth Letter) | Antitachycardia Functions (Fifth Letter) |
| O = None | O = None (fixed-rate pacemaker) | O = None (fixed-rate pacemaker) | O = None | O = None |
| A = Atrium | A = Atrium | T = Triggers pacing | P = Simple programmability (rate and/or output) | P = Pacing (antitachycardia) |
| V = Ventricle | V = Ventricle | I = Inhibits pacing | M = Multiprogrammable | S = Shock |
| D = Dual chamber (atrium and ventricle) | D = Dual chamber (atrium and ventricle) | D = Dual (triggers and inhibits pacing) | C = Communication | D = Dual (pacing and shock) |
| | | | R = Rate responsive | |

(Figure 8-3). Atrial pacing may be used when the SA node is diseased or damaged, but conduction through the AV junction and ventricles is normal. This type of pacemaker is ineffective if an AV block develops because it cannot pace the ventricles.

Ventricular pacing is accomplished by placing the pacing electrode in the right ventricle. Stimulation of the ventricles produces a pacemaker spike on the ECG followed by a wide QRS, resembling a ventricular ectopic beat (Figure 8-4). The QRS complex is wide because a paced impulse does not follow the normal conduction pathway in the heart.

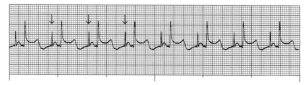

**Figure 8-3**   Atrial pacing.

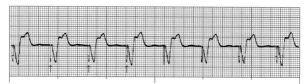

**Figure 8-4**   Ventricular pacing.

## Dual-Chamber Pacemakers

A pacemaker that paces both the atrium and ventricle has a two-lead system placed in the heart; one lead is placed in the right atrium, the other in the right ventricle. This type of pacemaker is called a dual-chamber pacemaker. An AV sequential pacemaker is an example of a dual-chamber pacemaker. The AV sequential pacemaker stimulates the right atrium and right ventricle sequentially (stimulating first the atrium, then the ventricle), mimicking normal cardiac physiology and thus preserving the atrial contribution to ventricular filling (atrial kick) (Figure 8-5).

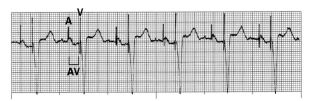

**Figure 8-5**  AV sequential pacing. *A,* atrial pacing, *V,* ventricular pacing, *AV,* AV interval.

## TRANSCUTANEOUS PACING (TCP)

### Indications

TCP is effective, quick, safe, and the least invasive pacing technique currently available. TCP is indicated for significant bradycardias unresponsive to atropine therapy or when atropine is not immediately available or indicated. It may also be used as a bridge until transvenous pacing can be accomplished or the cause of the bradycardia is reversed (as in cases of drug overdose or hyperkalemia).

The primary limitation of TCP is patient discomfort that is proportional to the intensity of skeletal muscle contraction and the direct electrical stimulation of cutaneous nerves. The degree of discomfort varies with the device used and the stimulating current required to achieve capture.

## PACEMAKER MALFUNCTION

### Failure to Pace

Failure to pace is a pacemaker malfunction that occurs when the pacemaker fails to deliver an electrical stimulus or when it fails to deliver the correct number of electrical stimulations per minute. Failure to pace is recognized on the ECG as an absence of pacemaker spikes (even though the patient's intrinsic rate is less than that of the pacemaker) and a return of the underlying rhythm for which the pacemaker was implanted. Patient signs and symptoms may include syncope, chest pain, bradycardia, and hypotension.

Treatment may include adjusting the sensitivity setting, replacing the pulse generator battery, replacing the pacing lead, replacing the pulse generator unit, tightening connections between the pacing lead and pulse generator, performing an electrical check, and/or removing the source of electromagnetic interference.

## Failure to Capture

Capture is successful depolarization of the atria and/or ventricles by an artificial pacemaker and is obtained after the pacemaker electrode is properly positioned in the heart. Failure to capture is the inability of the pacemaker stimulus to depolarize the myocardium and is recognized on the ECG by visible pacemaker spikes not followed by P waves (if the electrode is located in the atrium) or QRS complexes (if the electrode is located in the right ventricle) (Figure 8-6). Patient signs and symptoms may include fatigue, bradycardia, and hypotension. Treatment may include repositioning the patient, slowly increasing the output setting (mA) until capture occurs or the maximum setting is reached, replacing the pulse generator battery, replacing or repositioning of the pacing lead, or surgery.

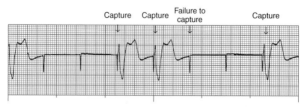

**Figure 8-6**   Failure to capture.

## Failure to Sense (Undersensing)

Sensitivity is the extent to which a pacemaker recognizes intrinsic electrical activity. Failure to sense occurs when the pacemaker fails to recognize spontaneous myocardial depolarization (Figure 8-7). This pacemaker malfunction is recognized on the ECG by pacemaker spikes that follow too closely behind the patient's QRS complexes (earlier than the programmed escape interval). Because pacemaker spikes occur when they should not, this type of pacemaker malfunction may result in pacemaker spikes that fall on T waves (R-on-T phenomenon) and/or competition between the pacemaker and the patient's own cardiac rhythm. The patient may complain of palpitations or skipped beats. R-on-T phenomenon may precipitate VT or VF. Treatment may include increasing the sensitivity setting, replacing the pulse generator battery, and/or replacing or repositioning the pacing lead.

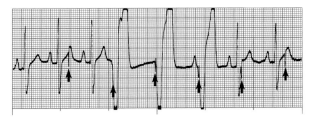

**Figure 8-7**   Failure to sense.

## Oversensing

Oversensing is a pacemaker malfunction that results from inappropriate sensing of extraneous electrical signals. Atrial sensing pacemakers may inappropriately sense ventricular activity; ventricular sensing pacemakers may misidentify a tall, peaked intrinsic T wave as a QRS complex. Oversensing is recognized on the ECG as pacemaker spikes at a rate slower than the pacemaker's preset rate (paced QRS complexes that come later than the pacemaker's preset escape interval) or no paced beats even though the pacemaker's preset rate is greater than the patient's intrinsic rate.

The patient with a pacemaker should avoid strong electro-magnetic fields such as those associated with welding equipment or a magnetic resonance imaging (MRI) machine. Treatment includes adjustment of the pacemaker's sensitivity setting or possible insertion of a bipolar lead if oversensing is caused by unipolar lead dysfunction.

## ANALYZING PACEMAKER FUNCTION ON THE ECG

### Identify the Intrinsic Rate and Rhythm

- Are P waves present? At what rate?
- Are QRS complexes present? At what rate?

### Is There Evidence of Paced Activity?

- If paced atrial activity is present, evaluate the paced interval.
- Using calipers or paper, measure the distance between two consecutively paced atrial beats.
- Determine the rate and regularity of the paced interval.
- If paced ventricular activity is present, evaluate the paced interval.
- Using calipers or paper, measure the distance between two consecutively paced ventricular beats.
- Determine the rate and regularity of the paced interval.

### Evaluate the Escape Interval

- Compare the escape interval to the paced interval measured earlier. The paced interval and escape interval should measure the same.

### Analyze the Rhythm Strip

- Analyze the rhythm strip for failure to capture, failure to sense, oversensing, and failure to pace.

# Introduction to the 12-Lead ECG

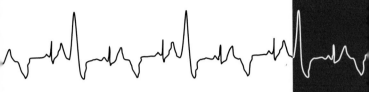

## INTRODUCTION TO THE 12-LEAD ECG

A standard 12-lead ECG provides views of the heart in both the frontal and horizontal planes and views the surfaces of the left ventricle from 12 different angles. Multiple views of the heart can provide useful information including:

- Recognition of bundle branch blocks
- Identification of ST-segment and T wave changes associated with myocardial ischemia, injury, and infarction
- Identification of ECG changes associated with certain medications and electrolyte imbalances

Indications for using a 12-lead ECG include the following:

- Chest pain or discomfort
- Assisting in dysrhythmia interpretation
- Right and/or left ventricular failure
- Status before and after electrical therapy (defibrillation, cardioversion, pacing)
- Syncope or near syncope
- Electrical injuries
- Stroke
- Known or suspected medication overdoses
- Known or suspected electrolyte imbalances

## VECTORS

Leads have a negative (−) and positive (+) electrode pole that senses the magnitude and direction of the electrical force caused by the spread of waves of depolarization and repolarization throughout the myocardium. A vector (arrow) is a symbol representing this force. Leads that face the tip or point of a vector record a positive deflection on ECG paper.

A mean vector identifies the average of depolarization waves in one portion of the heart. The mean P vector represents the average magnitude and direction of both right and left atrial depolarization. The mean QRS vector represents the average magnitude and direction of both right and left ventricular depolarization. The average direction of a mean vector is called the mean axis and is only identified in the frontal plane. An imaginary line joining the positive and negative electrodes of a lead is called the axis of the lead. Electrical axis refers to determining the direction (or angle in degrees) in which the main vector of depolarization is pointed.

### Axis

During normal ventricular depolarization, the left side of the interventricular septum is stimulated first. The electrical impulse then traverses the septum to stimulate the right side. The left and right ventricles are then depolarized simultaneously. Because the left ventricle is considerably larger than the right, right ventricular depolarization forces are overshadowed on the ECG. As a result, the mean QRS vector points down (inferior) and to the left.

The axes of leads I, II, and III form an equilateral triangle with the heart at the center (Einthoven's triangle). If the augmented limb leads are added to this configuration and the axes of the six leads moved in a way in which they bisect each other, the result is the hexaxial reference system (Figure 9-1).

The hexaxial reference system represents all of the frontal plane (limb) leads with the heart in the center and is the means used to express the location of the frontal plane axis.

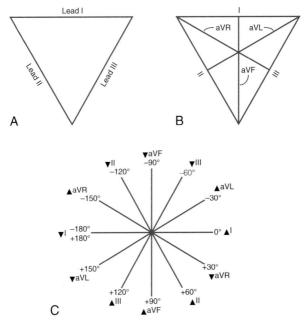

**Figure 9-1 A-C, A,** Einthoven's equilateral triangle formed by leads I, II, and III. **B,** The unipolar leads are added to the equilateral triangle. **C,** The hexaxial reference system derived from **B.**

This system forms a 360-degree circle surrounding the heart. The positive end of lead I is designated at 0 degrees. The six frontal plane leads divide the circle into segments, each representing 30 degrees. All degrees in the upper hemisphere are labeled as negative degrees, and all degrees in the lower hemisphere are labeled as positive degrees. The mean QRS vector (normal electrical axis) lies between 0 and +90 degrees.

Current flow to the right of normal is called right axis deviation (+90 to +180 degrees). Current flow in the direction opposite of normal is called indeterminate, "no man's land," northwest or extreme right axis deviation ($-91$ to $-179$ degrees). Current flow to the left of normal is called left axis deviation ($-1$ to $-90$ degrees).

Leads I and aVF divide the heart into four quadrants. These two leads can be used to quickly estimate electrical axis. In leads I and aVF, the QRS complex is normally positive. If the QRS complex in either or both of these leads is negative, axis deviation is present (Table 9-1).

| Table **9-1** | Two-Lead Method of Axis Determination | | | |
|---|---|---|---|---|
| Axis | Normal | Left | Right | Indeterminate ("No Man's Land") |
| Lead I – QRS Direction | Positive | Positive | Negative | Negative |
| Lead aVF – QRS Direction | Positive | Negative | Positive | Negative |

## LAYOUT OF THE 12-LEAD ECG

Most 12-lead monitors record all 12 leads simultaneously but display them in a conventional 3-row by 4-column format. The standard limb leads are recorded in the first column, the augmented limb leads in the second column, and the chest leads in the third and fourth columns. All of the QRS complexes in a row are consecutive while QRS complexes that are aligned vertically represent a simultaneous recording of the same beat. Because the leads are obtained simultaneously, only 10 seconds of sampling time is required to record all twelve leads

## ACUTE CORONARY SYNDROMES

Acute coronary syndromes (ACS) are conditions caused by a similar sequence of pathologic events—a temporary or permanent blockage of a coronary artery. This sequence of events results in conditions ranging from myocardial ischemia or injury to death (necrosis) of heart muscle. ACS include unstable angina, non–ST-segment elevation MI (NSTEMI), and ST-segment elevation MI (STEMI). Sudden cardiac death can occur with any of these conditions. The usual cause of an ACS is the rupture of an atherosclerotic plaque.

## LOCALIZATION OF INFARCTIONS

### Contiguous Leads

When ECG changes of myocardial ischemia, injury, or infarction occur, they are not found in every lead of the ECG. Findings are considered significant if viewed in two or more leads looking at the same area of the heart. If these findings are seen in leads that look directly at the affected area, they are called indicative changes. If findings are seen in leads opposite the affected area, they are called reciprocal changes (also called "mirror image" changes) (Figure 9-2). Of the indicative changes, ST-segment elevation provides the strongest evidence for the early recognition of MI. ST-segment elevation is considered significant when it is elevated at least 1 mm and is viewed in two or more leads looking at the same area of the heart.

Indicative changes are significant when they are seen in two anatomically contiguous leads. Two leads are contiguous if they look at the same area of the heart or they are numerically consecutive chest leads. Table 9-2 shows the area viewed by each lead of a standard 12-lead ECG.

| Table **9-2** | Localizing ECG Changes | | | | |
|---|---|---|---|---|---|
| I | Lateral | aVR — | V1 septum | V4 anterior | V4R right ventricle |
| II | Inferior | aVL lateral | V2 septum | V5 lateral | V5R right ventricle |
| III | Inferior | aVF inferior | V3 anterior | V6 lateral | V6R right ventricle |

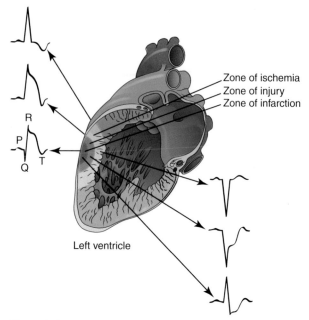

Zone of ischemia
Zone of injury
Zone of infarction

Left ventricle

**Figure 9-2** Zones of ischemia, injury, and infarction showing indicative ECG changes and reciprocal changes corresponding to each zone.

## PREDICTING THE SITE AND EXTENT OF CORONARY ARTERY OCCLUSION

Since myocardial infarction is the result of an occluded coronary artery, it is worthwhile to develop a familiarity with the coronary arteries that supply the heart. Once the infarction has been recognized and localized, an understanding of coronary artery anatomy makes it possible to predict which coronary artery is occluded.

In the standard 12-lead ECG, leads II, III, and aVF "look" at tissue supplied by the right coronary artery and eight leads "look" at tissue supplied by the left coronary artery—leads I, aVL, $V_1$, $V_2$, $V_3$, $V_4$, $V_5$, and $V_6$. When evaluating the extent of infarction produced by a left coronary artery occlusion, determine how many of these leads are showing changes consistent with an acute infarction. The more of these eight leads demonstrating acute changes, the larger the infarction is presumed to be.

To identify the site of occlusion, compare the infarct location with the coronary anatomy. If an ECG shows changes in leads II, III, and aVF, suspect an inferior wall infarction. Since the inferior wall of the left ventricle is supplied by the right coronary artery in most of the population, it is reasonable to suppose that this infarct is due to a right coronary artery occlusion. When indicative changes are seen in the leads viewing the septal, anterior, and/or lateral walls of the left ventricle ($V_1$-$V_6$, I, and aVL), it is reasonable to suspect a left coronary artery occlusion. Table 9-3 summarizes the pattern in which coronary arteries most commonly supply the myocardium.

## INTRAVENTRICULAR CONDUCTION DELAYS

### Bundle Branch Activation

During normal ventricular depolarization, the left side of the interventricular septum (stimulated by the left posterior fascicle) is stimulated first. The electrical impulse (wave of depolarization) then traverses the septum to stimulate the right side. The left and right ventricles are then depolarized at the same time. If a delay or block occurs in one of the bundle branches, the ventricles will not be depolarized at the same time. The impulse first travels down the unblocked branch and stimulates that ventricle. Because of the block, the impulse must then travel from cell to cell through the myocardium (rather than through the normal conduction pathway) to stimulate the other ventricle. This means of conduction is slower than normal, and the QRS complex appears widened

**Table 9-3    Localization of a Myocardial Infarction**

| Location of MI | Indicative Changes (Leads Facing Affected Area) | Reciprocal Changes (Leads Opposite Affected Area) | Affected Coronary Artery |
|---|---|---|---|
| Anterior | $V_3$, $V_4$ | $V_7$, $V_8$, $V_9$ | Left coronary artery<br>• LAD – diagonal branch |
| Anteroseptal | $V_1$, $V_2$, $V_3$, $V_4$ | $V_7$, $V_8$, $V_9$ | Left coronary artery<br>• LAD – diagonal branch<br>• LAD – septal branch |
| Anterolateral | I, aVL, $V_3$, $V_4$, $V_5$, $V_6$ | II, III, aVF, $V_7$, $V_8$, $V_9$ | Left coronary artery<br>• LAD – diagonal branch and/or<br>Circumflex branch |
| Inferior | II, III, aVF | I, aVL | Right coronary artery (most common) – posterior descending branch or Left coronary artery – circumflex branch |
| Lateral | I, aVL, $V_5$, $V_6$ | II, III, aVF | Left coronary artery<br>• LAD – diagonal branch and/or<br>Circumflex branch<br>Right coronary artery |
| Septum | $V_1$, $V_2$ | $V_7$, $V_8$, $V_9$ | Left coronary artery<br>• LAD – septal branch |
| Posterior | $V_7$, $V_8$, $V_9$ | $V_1$, $V_2$, $V_3$ | Right coronary or circumflex artery |
| Right Ventricle | $V_1R$-$V_6R$ | I, aVL | Right coronary artery<br>• Proximal branches |

on the ECG. The ventricle with the blocked bundle branch is the last to be depolarized.

Following are ECG criteria for identification of a right or left bundle branch block (BBB):

- QRS duration of more than 0.12 second (if a complete BBB)
- QRS complexes produced by supraventricular activity (i.e., the QRS complex is not a paced beat, and it did not originate in the ventricles)

When measuring for BBB, select the widest QRS complex with a discernible beginning and end. Lead $V_1$ is probably the single best lead to use when differentiating between right and left BBB.

A QRS measuring 0.10 to 0.12 second is called an incomplete right or left BBB. A QRS measuring more than 0.12 second is called a complete right or left BBB. If the QRS is wide but no BBB pattern is discernable, the term wide QRS or intraventricular conduction delay is used to describe the QRS.

Examination of the terminal force (final portion) of the QRS complex reveals the ventricle that was depolarized last, and therefore the bundle that was blocked. To identify the terminal force, first look at lead $V_1$ and locate the J point. Move from the J point backward into the QRS complex and determine if the terminal portion (last 0.04 sec) of the QRS complex is a positive (upright) or negative (downward) deflection (Figure 9-3). If it is directed upward, a right BBB is present (the current is moving toward the right ventricle and toward $V_1$). A left BBB is present when the terminal force of the QRS complex is directed downward (the current is moving away from $V_1$ and toward the left ventricle). A simple way to remember this rule is demonstrated in Figure 9-4. As shown in the figure, this rule is similar to the turn indicator on a vehicle. When a right turn is made, the turn indicator is lifted up. Likewise, when a right BBB is present, the terminal force of the QRS complex

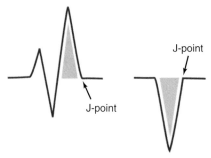

**Figure 9-3**   Move from the J point back into the QRS complex and determine if the terminal portion (last 0.04 second) of the QRS complex is a positive (upright) or negative (downward) deflection. If the two criteria for bundle branch block are met and the terminal portion of the QRS is positive, a RBBB is most likely present. If the terminal portion of the QRS is negative, a LBBB is most likely present.

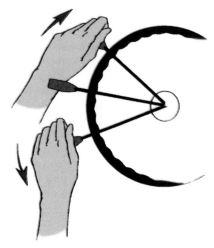

**Figure 9-4**   Differentiating right versus left BBB. The "turn signal theory"— right is up, left is down.

points up. Conversely, left turns and left BBB are directed downward.

Two notable exceptions must be mentioned to complete the discussion of BBB. The first involves the criteria used to recognized BBB, while the second relates to differentiating LBBB from RBBB. The criteria used to recognize BBB are valid, but lack some sensitivity and specificity. The sensitivity can be limited by junctional rhythms because there may be no discernible P waves when the AV junction is the pacemaker site. While the AV junction is a supraventricular pacemaker, this presents as an exception to the two-part rule of BBB recognition. Specificity is limited by Wolff-Parkinson-White syndrome (WPW) and other conditions that produce wide QRS complexes resulting from atrial activity. If the characteristic delta wave and shortened PR interval are recognized, then WPW can be suspected. Similarly, hyperkalemia and other conditions that can widen the QRS are relatively infrequent

## CHAMBER ENLARGEMENT

Enlargement of the atrial and/or ventricular chambers of the heart may occur if there is a volume or pressure overload in the heart. Dilatation is an increase in the diameter of a chamber of the heart caused by volume overload. Dilatation may be acute or chronic. Hypertrophy is an increase in the thickness of a heart chamber because of chronic pressure overload. Enlargement is a term that implies the presence of dilatation or hypertrophy or both.

### Atrial Enlargement

The first half of the P wave is recorded when the electrical impulse that originated in the SA node stimulates the right atrium and reaches the AV node. The downslope of the P wave reflects stimulation of the left atrium. A normal P wave is smooth and rounded, no more than 2.5 mm in height, and no more than 0.11 sec in duration (width). Normal P waves are positive (upright) in leads I, II, aVF, and $V_4$ through $V_6$.

## Right Atrium

Enlargement of the right atrium produces an abnormally tall initial part of the P wave. The P wave is tall (2.5 mm or more in height in leads II, III, and aVF), peaked, and of normal duration. This type of P wave is called P pulmonale because right atrial enlargement (RAE) is usually caused by conditions that increase the work of the right atrium, such as chronic obstructive pulmonary disease with or without pulmonary hypertension, congenital heart disease, or right ventricular failure of any cause.

## Left Atrium

The latter part of the P wave is prominent in left atrial enlargement (LAE). This is because the impulse starts in the right atrium where the SA node is located and chamber size is normal. The electrical impulse then travels to the left to depolarize the left atrium. The waveform inscribed on the ECG is widened (latter part of the P wave) because it takes longer to depolarize an enlarged muscle. The P wave is more than 0.11 sec in duration and often notched in leads I, II, aVL, and $V_4$, $V_5$, and $V_6$.

## Ventricular Enlargement

Ventricular muscle thickens (hypertrophies) when it sustains a persistent pressure overload. Dilatation occurs because of persistent volume overload. The two often go hand in hand. Hypertrophy increases the QRS amplitude and is often associated with ST-segment depression and asymmetric T wave inversion. The ST-segment depression and T wave inversion pattern is called *ventricular strain* or *secondary repolarization changes*.

## Right Ventricle

Because the right ventricle is normally considerably smaller than the left, it must become extremely enlarged before changes are visible on the ECG. Right axis deviation is one of the earliest and most reliable findings of right ventricular hypertrophy (RVH). Further, normal R wave progression is reversed in the chest leads, revealing taller than normal R waves and small S waves in $V_1$ and $V_2$ and deeper than normal S waves and small R waves in $V_5$ and $V_6$.

### Left Ventricle

Recognition of left ventricular hypertrophy (LVH) on the ECG is not always obvious, and many methods to assist in its recognition have been suggested. ECG signs of LVH include deeper than normal S waves and small R waves in $V_1$ and $V_2$ and taller than normal R waves and small S waves in $V_5$ and $V_6$. If S wave amplitude in lead $V_1$ added to the R wave amplitude in $V_5$ is greater than or equal to 35 mV, LVH should be suspected. Causes of LVH include systemic hypertension, hypertrophic cardiomyopathy, aortic stenosis, and aortic insufficiency. LVH may be accompanied by left axis deviation.

## ECG CHANGES ASSOCIATED WITH ELECTROLYTE DISTURBANCES

A summary of the ECG changes associated with electrolyte disturbances can be found in Table 9-4.

## ANALYZING THE 12-LEAD ECG

When analyzing a 12-lead ECG, it is important to use a systematic method. Begin by assessing the quality of the tracing. If baseline wander or artifact is present to any significant degree, note it. If the presence of either of these conditions interferes with the assessment of any lead, use a modifier such as "possible" or "apparent" in your interpretation. Next, identify the rate and underlying rhythm. Evaluate intervals— PR interval, QRS duration, and the QT interval and then evaluate waveforms—P waves, Q waves, R waves (R wave progression), T waves, and U waves. If a Q wave is present, express the duration in milliseconds. Examine each lead for the presence of ST-segment displacement (elevation or depression). If ST-segment elevation is present, express it in

**Table 9-4** ECG Changes Associated with Electrolyte Disturbances

| Electrolyte Disturbance | P Wave | PR Interval | QRS Complex | ST-Segment | T Wave | QT Interval | Heart Rate |
|---|---|---|---|---|---|---|---|
| Hypocalcemia | | | | Long, flattened | | Prolonged | |
| Hypercalcemia | | | | Shortened | | Shortened | |
| Hypokalemia | | Prolonged | Widen as level decreases | Depressed | Flattened; U wave present | Prolonged | |
| Hyperkalemia | Disappear as level increases | Normal or prolonged | Widen as level increases | Disappear as level increases | Tall, peaked or tented | | Slows |
| Hypomagnesemia | Diminished voltage (amplitude) | | Widen as level decreases; diminished voltage | Depressed | Flattened; U wave present | Prolonged | |
| Hypermagnesemia | | Prolonged | Widened | | Tall or elevated | | |

millimeters. Assess the areas of ischemia or injury by assessing lead groupings. Examine the T waves for any changes in orientation, shape, and size.

Determine axis, look for evidence of hypertrophy/chamber enlargement, and look for effects of medications and electrolyte imbalances. Interpret your findings.

# Credits

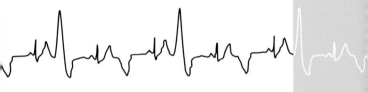

## CHAPTER 1

**Figure 1-1**   Herlihy B, Maebius NK: *The human body in health and illness,* ed 3, St Louis, 2007, WB Saunders.

**Figure 1-2**   Thibodeau GA, Patton KT: *Anatomy and physiology,* ed 7, St Louis, 2010, Mosby.

**Figure 1-3**   Drake, R, Vogl W, Mitchell, A: *Gray's anatomy for students,* ed 2, Philadelphia, 2010, Churchill Livingstone.

**Figure 1-5**   Herlihy B, Maebius NK: *The human body in health and illness,* ed 3, St Louis, 2007, WB Saunders.

## CHAPTER 2

**Figure 2-1**   Thibodeau GA, Patton KT: *Anatomy and physiology,* ed 7, St Louis, 2010, Mosby.

**Figure 2-2, 2-3, 2-4**   Herlihy B, Maebius NK: *The human body in health and illness,* ed 3, St Louis, 2007, WB Saunders.

**Figure 2-5**   Sanders MJ: *Mosby's paramedic textbook,* St Louis, 1994, Mosby.

**Figure 2-6**   Thelan LA, Davie JK, Urden LD, Lough ME: *Critical care nursing: diagnosis and management,* ed 2, St Louis, 1993, Mosby.

**Figure 2-7**   Crawford MV, Spence MI: *Common sense approach to coronary care,* revised ed 6, St Louis, 1994, Mosby.

**Figure 2-8**    Herlihy B, Maebius NK: *The human body in health and illness,* ed 3, St Louis, 2007, WB Saunders.

**Figure 2-9**    Goldberger A: *Clinical electrocardiography: a simplified approach,* ed 6, St Louis, 1998, Mosby.

**Figure 2-10**    Urden LD, Stacy KM, Lough ME: *Thelans's critical care nursing: diagnosis and management,* ed 5, St Louis, 2006, Mosby.

**Figure 2-11**    Goldberger A: *Clinical electrocardiography: a simplified approach,* ed 6, St Louis, 1998, Mosby.

**Figure 2-12**    Thelan LA, Davie JK, Urden LD, Lough ME: *Critical care nursing: diagnosis and management,* ed 2, St Louis, 1993, Mosby.

**Figure 2-13**    Thibodeau GA, Patton KT: *Anatomy and physiology,* ed 7, St Louis, 2010, Mosby.

**Figure 2-15, 2-16, 2-17**    Modified from Noble A, Johnson R, Thomas A, & Bass P: *The cardiovascular system,* Philadelphia, 2005, Churchill Livingstone.

**Figure 2-20**    Urden LD, Stacy KM, Lough ME: *Thelans's critical care nursing: diagnosis and management,* ed 5, St Louis, 2006, Mosby.

**Figure 2-21**    Crawford MV, Spence MI: *Common sense approach to coronary care,* revised ed 6, St Louis, 1994, Mosby.

## CHAPTER 4

**Figure 4-2**    Kinney MP, Packa DR: *Andreoli's comprehensive cardiac care,* ed 8, St Louis, 1996, Mosby.

**Figure 4-4**    Goldberger A: *Clinical electrocardiography: a simplified approach,* ed 6, St Louis, 1998, Mosby.

**Figure 4-5**    Braunwald E, Zipes DP, Libby P: *Heart disease: a textbook of cardiovascular medicine,* ed 6, Philadelphia, 2001, WB Saunders.

**Figure 4-6**    Goldberger A: *Clinical electrocardiography: a simplified approach,* ed 6, St Louis, 1998, Mosby.

**Figure 4-7**    Shade B, Rothenberg M, Wertz E, Jones S, Collins T: *Mosby's EMT-Intermediate Textbook,* 2e, St. Louis, 2002, Mosby.

**Figure 4-9**    Urden LD, Stacy KM, Lough ME: *Thelans's critical care nursing: diagnosis and management,* ed 5, St Louis, 2006, Mosby.

**Figure 4-10** Goldberger A: *Clinical electrocardiography: a simplified approach*, ed 6, St Louis, 1998, Mosby.

**Figure 4-11** Grauer K: *A practical guide to ECG interpretation*, ed 2, St Louis, 1998, Mosby.

## CHAPTER 5

**Figures 5-2, 5-3** Grauer K: *A practical guide to ECG interpretation*, ed 2, St Louis, 1998, Mosby.

## CHAPTER 6

**Figure 6-1** Grauer K: *A practical guide to ECG interpretation*, ed 2, St Louis, 1998, Mosby.

**Figure 6-2** Kinney MP, Packa DR: *Andreoli's comprehensive cardiac care*, ed 8, St Louis, 1996, Mosby.

**Figure 6-8** Surawicz B, Knilans TK: *Chou's electrocardiography in clinical practice: adult and pediatric*, ed 5, Philadelphia, 1996, Saunders.

**Figure 6-11** Crawford MV, Spence MI: *Common sense approach to coronary care,* revised ed 6, St Louis, 1994, Mosby.

**Figure 6-17** Grauer K: *A practical guide to ECG interpretation*, ed 2, St Louis, 1998, Mosby.

## CHAPTER 7

**Figure 7-7** Grauer K: *A practical guide to ECG interpretation*, ed 2, St Louis, 1998, Mosby.

## CHAPTER 9

**Figure 9-1** Surawicz B, Knilans TK: *Chou's electrocardiography in clinical practice: adult and pediatric*, ed 5, Philadelphia, 1996, WB Saunders.

**Table 9-3, 9-4** Aehlert B: *Paramedic practice today*, St. Louis, 2010, Mosby.

# Index

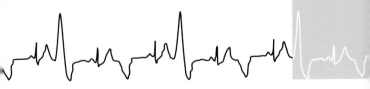